Face Exercises That Prevent Premature Aging

By Jeanette Johnson

Illustrated by Jeanette Johnson and Jade

Shipley Press - Dallas, Texas

Published by Shipley Press, Dallas, Texas

Typeset by Patty Arndt
carndt@ibm.net
Rochester, MN

ISBN 0-9647384-0-6
Library of Congress Catalog Card:95-92376

Before you begin using Designer Exercises
and the Skin-Smoothing Masque,
get your doctor's approval for your
use of these skin-care techniques.

Printed in the United States of America

Table of Contents

Introduction To Designer Exercises

About Designer Exercises

Designer Exercises are face exercises designed to prevent premature aging of the face. Premature aging happens because Father Time is still using the same aging clock he was using thousands of years ago when our ancestors lived less than half the years that women and men can now expect to live.

Modern medicine and good health practices have lengthened the life span so dramatically that people are young adults until age 45 or 50. Then come youthful middle years that can last indefinitely. Looking older than you are makes no sense and Designer Exercises can help you prevent it.

A Note to the Reader from Jeanette Johnson

Over thirty years ago I began inventing Designer Exercises and I have used them to escape an aging prediction made to me when I was a child. I was the ugly duckling in a family that placed high value on beauty; I was the kid with the big ears, crooked teeth, and splotchy freckles. Compared to the rest of the gang, I placed last when it came to looks. Worse yet, I was told I had inherited the kind of skin that was going to "wrinkle early". Ouch! That "wrinkle early" prediction meant my fate was to be, not only ugly, but old before my time. The more I thought about this, the less I liked it and I made up my mind that somehow I would find a way to make that prediction a false one.

As the years passed, I studied people's faces to find out what happened to the skin to make it look older. I learned that signs of aging begin to show in almost everybody's face before they have their 35th birthday and realized I was not the only person at risk for premature aging. Lines and sags appear much too soon in the faces of both women and men.

This seemed a cruel fate and I became even more determined to find a way to change it. My search for a way to prevent premature aging culminated in the invention of Designer Exercises for the face and a Skin-Smoothing Masque for the face and hands.

These exercises are called Designer Exercises because each one is designed for a specific area of the face and because I wanted them to be known as a special kind of exercises. Designer Exercises and the Skin-Smoothing Masque enabled me to escape the "wrinkle early" prediction. At age 64, I am still using these skin-care techniques and they are still working for me.

My inspiration through the years was a beautiful princess who became Queen of England in 1901 after the death of Queen Victoria. This princess kept her youthful looks as long as she lived. Her story provides an example of how the avoidance of premature aging can affect your life. To read about her, turn the page.

Alexandra, Princess of Wales

Alexandra was a remarkable woman who, I believe, used face exercises to keep her beauty throughout her life. She married Edward, Prince of Wales, when she was eighteen. He was Queen Victoria's oldest son. Almost forty years later when Alexandra became queen, she was as beautiful as she had been on her wedding day. The many photographs taken of her show that she changed very little as she grew older. When she was crowned queen at age 57, she had the face and body of a young woman.

Alexandra's life with the prince gave her strong motivation to keep her youthful looks. Edward had been reluctant to marry and did so under pressure from his mother. Not long after the wedding, the prince embarked on a life-long career as a womanizer.

Queen Victoria arranged her son's marriage in an attempt to keep him respectable. She was concerned about his one-night stand with an actress that took place before he graduated from college.

During a summer vacation the prince went on military maneuvers. His governor accompanied him and guarded him closely. Edward's fellow officers noticed that he was not allowed the freedom they enjoyed and they felt sorry for him. One night they smuggled an actress into his room and Edward gratefully took advantage of this opportunity to have his first sexual experience with a woman.

When Queen Victoria heard about her son's night with the actress, she decided he needed a wife. She was confident that Edward would settle into a life of high moral character after he married. She failed to anticipate the opportunities marriage would provide him.

After his wedding, the prince no longer had to live at the palace under his mother's watchful eye. In addition, parliament voted him an income that enabled him to become a well-to-do philanderer.

A Mistress, And Face Exercises

Edward, Prince of Wales, and Lillie Langtry, his Mistress

Lillie Langtry was Edward's first publicly acknowledged mistress. Lillie met the prince not long after she made her entrance into London society where her beauty and wit gained her the attentions of many men. Oscar Wilde compared her to Helen of Troy. James Whistler marveled at her beauty and said he could not do justice to her in a painting.

Alexandra befriended her husband's celebrated mistress and when Lillie became pregnant, the princess was kind to her despite speculation that Edward was the child's father. Rumors that he had gotten Lillie pregnant embarrassed the prince and his affair with her came to an end.

To support herself and her child, Lillie studied acting and became an internationally known performer. She toured the United States and met Judge Roy Bean who named a town in Texas after her. When asked by American reporters how she managed to look ten years younger than her age of thirty-three, Lillie said physical exercise was her secret.

Lillie tried hard to keep her beauty. In an interview at age 49, she said she exercised an hour every morning. It is believed that her favorite exercise was jogging. Nevertheless, in middle age, the lovely Lillie began to fade. She declared with bitterness at 57 that she did not look at all young anymore. If Alexandra did face exercises, it seems that she did not share her beauty secret with Lillie.

The aging of her face caused Lillie much unhappiness. Her second husband was years younger than she and he paid little attention to her. When she died, he did not even attend her funeral.

Alexandra's husband, by contrast, remained her admirer. After his affair with Lillie ended, the Prince of Wales had a succession of lady loves but he had learned to care deeply for his wife. He was in awe of her lasting beauty and he was proud of her. He demonstrated his affection by refusing to allow an unkind or disrespectful remark to be made about her in his presence.

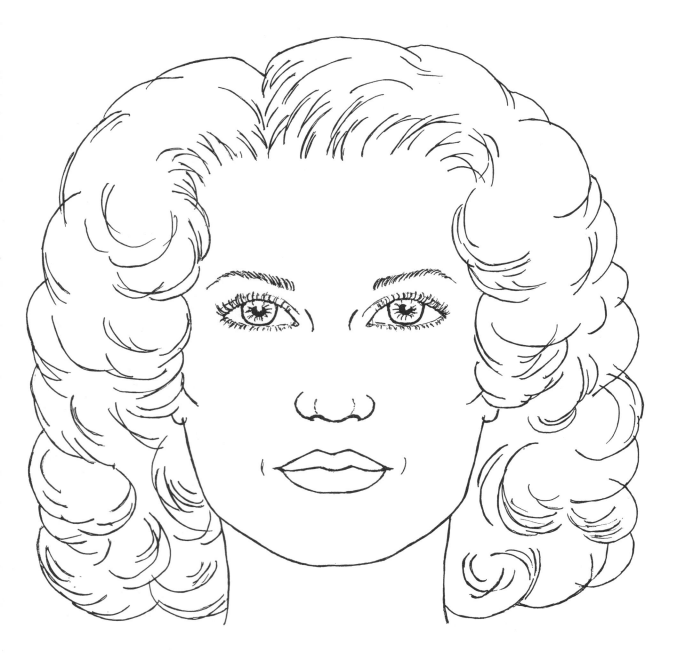

Premature Aging
What It Is ~ and Why It Happens

Before premature aging begins, muscles of the face are strong and tight. Both the muscles and underlying facial tissues have a fullness that serves as a supportive foundation for the skin.

Before one's 30th birthday, facial muscles begin losing strength as their elasticity and fullness diminish. This deterioration happens slowly but it continues with the passage of time.

A gradual shrinkage in the size of facial tissues also takes place. Fatty tissues around the muscles are particularly vulnerable; individual fat cells grow smaller and some are carried away as waste products of the body.

Without the support of strong muscles and healthy fatty tissues, the skin begins to develop premature aging signs.

Squint lines appear, cheeks sag, and flabbiness forms in the lower face. The mouth muscle grows thin and weak and this contributes to turn-in of the lips.

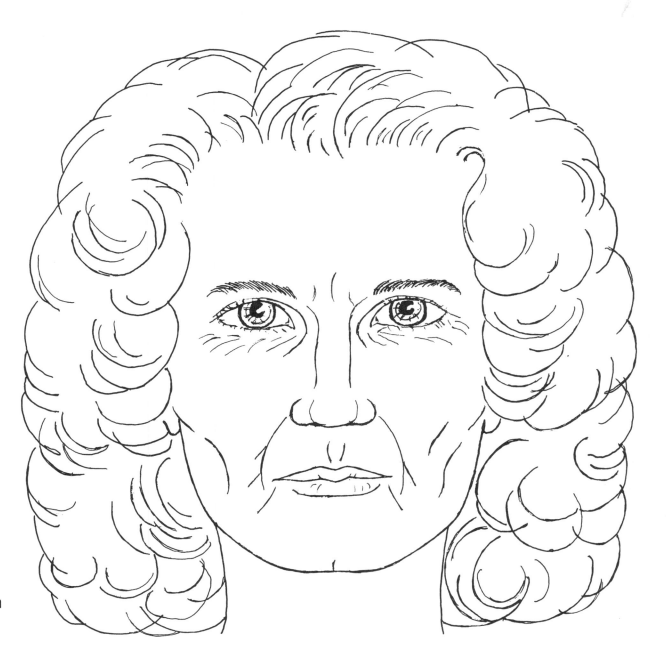

11

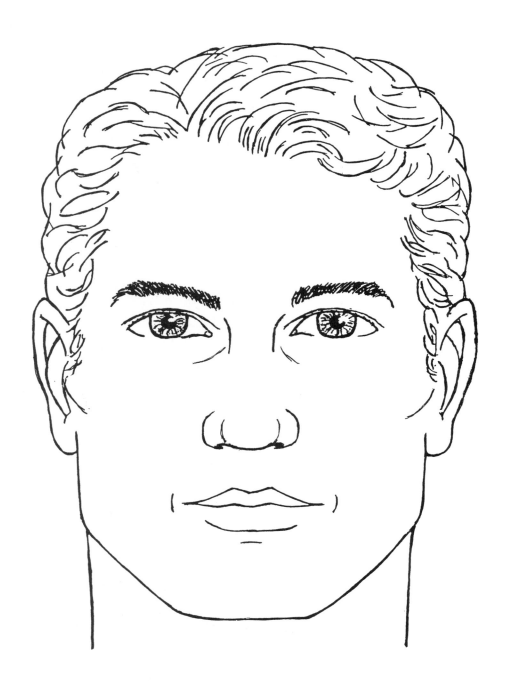

Men, Exercise and Premature Aging

Men have traditionally valued exercise as a way to keep their muscles strong so their bodies will stay in shape. They know that exercise can keep the body looking good so that its appearance doesn't change much as time passes. Many men prevent premature aging of their bodies by doing exercises that keep their body muscles strong.

Although exercising the body muscles makes a man look good

and feel good, it doesn't prevent a loss of strength and size in the muscles of his face.

Most men have thicker and tougher skin and muscles than women. This can make the premature aging process happen to a man's skin at a slower rate than it happens to a woman's skin.

Nevertheless, deterioration of the facial muscles and tissues eventually takes place and it detracts from the beauty of a man's face.

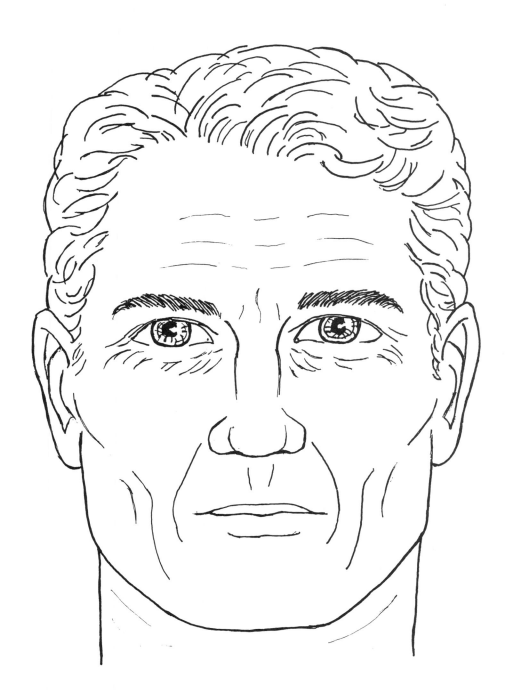

Muscles of the Face

The muscles in the illustration are the ones you will be using most in Designer Exercises.

The scientific names of the muscles are not used because they are difficult and you don't have to know them to do Designer Exercises. The muscles are called what they are: the eye, cheek, forehead, jaw, mouth, chin, and neck muscles.

Observe in the illustration how the muscles are made up of individual fibers. Each fiber is actually a long cell with intelligence of its own.

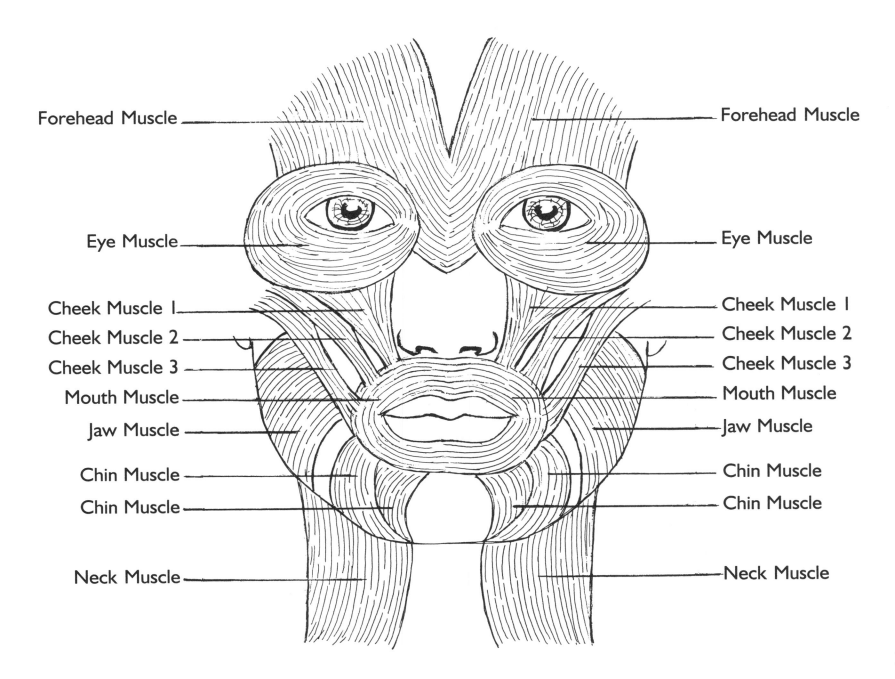

Forehead Muscle

Eye Muscle

Cheek Muscle 1
Cheek Muscle 2
Cheek Muscle 3
Mouth Muscle
Jaw Muscle

Chin Muscle
Chin Muscle

Neck Muscle

Forehead Muscle

Eye Muscle

Cheek Muscle 1
Cheek Muscle 2
Cheek Muscle 3
Mouth Muscle
Jaw Muscle

Chin Muscle
Chin Muscle

Neck Muscle

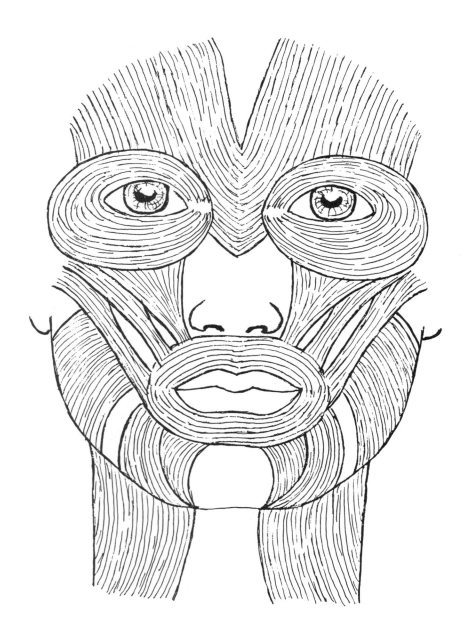

Before Premature Aging

The illustrations show the contrast between facial muscles before and after premature aging.

In the illustration on the left, the muscles are strong and tight. They support the skin around the eyes and the contours of the cheeks, lips, and lower face.

Notice how the cheek muscles insert into the mouth muscle and provide support for it.

After Premature Aging

Prematurely aged eye muscles are too weak to hold the skin firmly in place. This causes squint lines, hollows, and bags to form in the skin around the eyes.

In addition, cheek muscles sag and no longer provide support for the cheeks and the mouth muscle. When the mouth muscle lacks the support of strong cheek and chin muscles, the lips tend to turn inward.

Jaw and neck muscles become limp and slack and the skin attached to them becomes loose and shapeless.

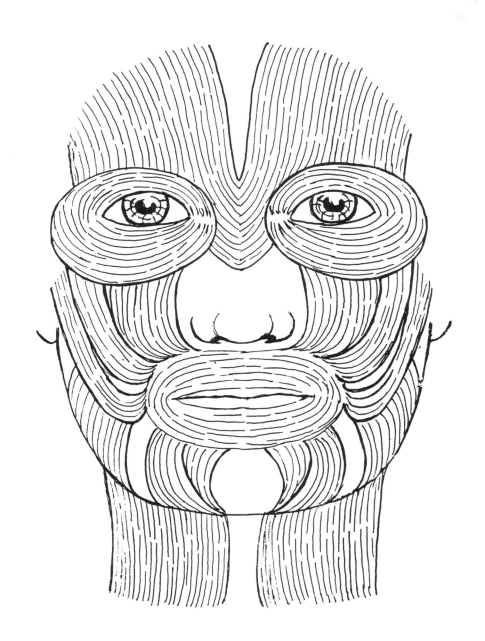

Muscles of the Face
and Their Routine Exercises

Muscles of the face are controlled by the will. The will is the signal you send from your brain to a muscle when you want the muscle to do something. Muscles contract and relax in response to the will.

When a muscle contracts, it shortens. This exerts a pull that can stretch another muscle. Since muscles have elasticity, they can return to their normal length after they are shortened or stretched.

For example, cheek muscles have their origin in the cheek bone and they are attached to the mouth muscle. When cheek muscles contract, they shorten and this raises the upper mouth muscle.

To observe this, look in a mirror, smile, and watch how the shortened cheek muscles raise your upper lip. Notice how your mouth muscle is stretched by the smile and observe how its elasticity returns it to its normal length after the smile.

Facial muscles get a measure of exercise when you smile, frown, squint, pucker your lips, or open your eyes. Nevertheless, these routine tasks do not provide the kind of exercise that strengthens the muscles. It is muscle activity that is much like the type of exercise you get when you go shopping; the exercise you get from doing this routine chore does not keep your body in shape.

By the same token, the exercise the face gets when its muscles do routine chores - does not keep the face in shape. It puts wear and tear on the muscles and the skin and contributes to premature aging.

Muscles of the face can shorten and stretch and then return to their normal length because of their elasticity. After about thirty years of life, they gradually and progressively lose elasticity. Eventually, they no longer have the strength to return to their original length after being stretched or shortened.

Squint lines are an example of what happens when a muscle has lost some of its elasticity. When the eye muscle squints, it contracts toward the nose and pulls the under-eye skin along with it.

Eventually, after thousands and thousands of squints, the muscle lacks sufficient elasticity and strength to return to its former length. Both muscle and skin remain stretched toward the nose and squint lines result.

Squint Contractions and Squint Consequences are illustrated on page 60 and 61.

Designer Exercises differ greatly from routine exercises done by the face. They build and strengthen the facial muscles. This helps prevent squint lines and many other signs of premature aging.

Designer Exercises provide an additional benefit; they stimulate the growth of fat cells around the muscles and this helps prevent the flat look that skin can acquire when it ages prematurely.

Premature aging detracts from the appearance of the face but its most devastating effect is on the lips and lower face. Sagging cheeks, turn-in of the lips and flabbiness in the jaws makes the entire face look older.

For this reason, the first Designer Exercises target these important areas of the face.

In each exercise I have included in the instructions the number of times for you to do the exercise daily. However, you can decide to do any exercise for longer periods of time if the muscle needs additional strengthening.

It would be difficult to do all of the exercises in the book every day, so you may want to do some of them each day and others two or three times weekly. In a problem area of the face you might choose to spend all of your time, for two or three days, exercising the muscles in this part of the face.

Designer Exercises For the Lips and Lower Face

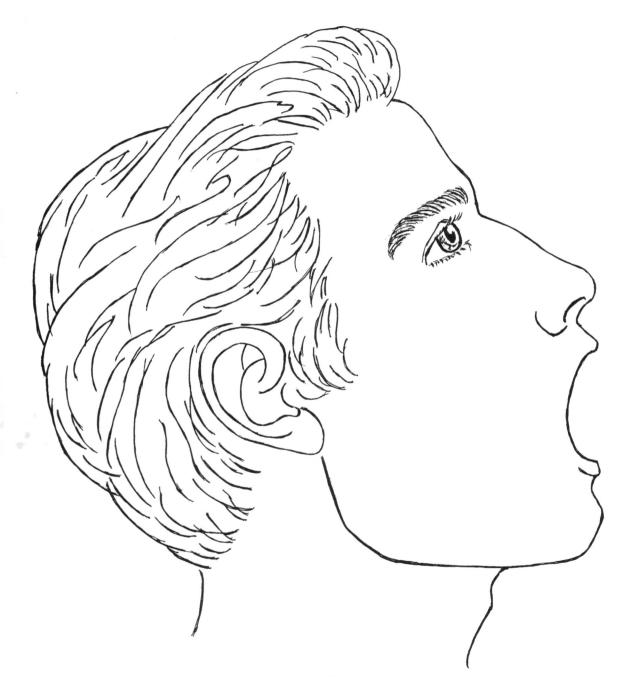

An Exercise For The Lips

1. Tilt your head back and open your mouth widely.

2. Bring your head back to its normal position and close your mouth.

3. Bring your chin forward as far as you can do so comfortably. This involves moving your jaw forward; no movement of the neck is involved.

4. Hold your chin and jaw forward to a count of five.

And The Mouth Muscle

5. Relax chin and jaw.

6. Bring your chin and jaw forward and push your closed lips forward without puckering them.

7. Hold lips flat together to a count of eight.

8. Relax lips, chin, and jaw.

Do exercise three times daily.

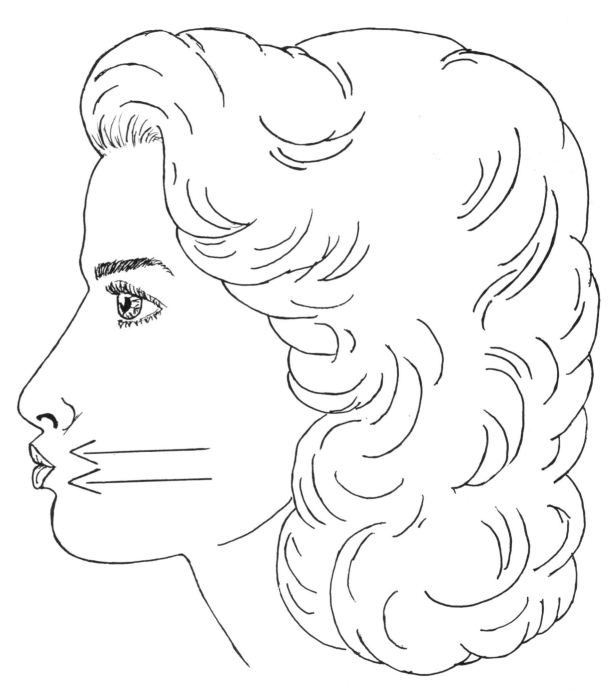

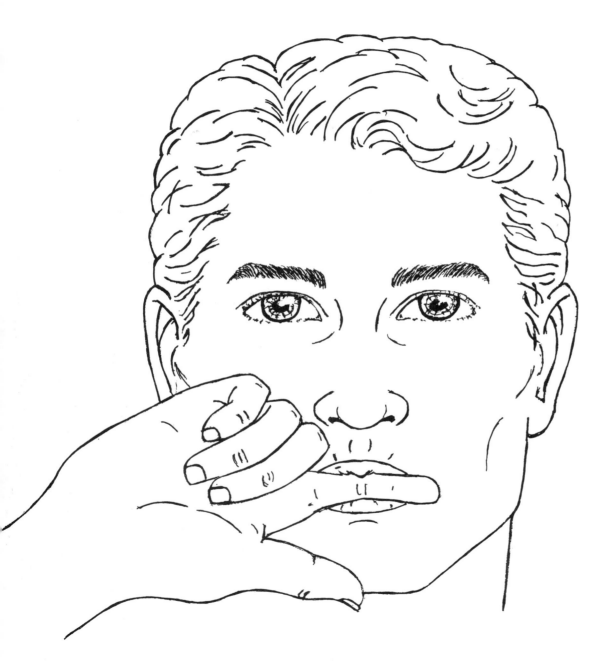

Exercises For the Lips and Mouth Muscle

Exercise One

1. Place the knuckle of your forefinger between your lips.

2. Take a deep breath and squeeze the knuckle with both lips to a count of four. Exhale as you squeeze the lips.

Do the exercise three to six times daily.

Exercise Two

1. Place the knuckle of your forefinger between your lips so the knuckle touches your teeth and your lips extend over the finger.

2. Take a deep breath and squeeze the knuckle with both lips to a count of five. Exhale as you count.

Do the exercise three or four times daily.

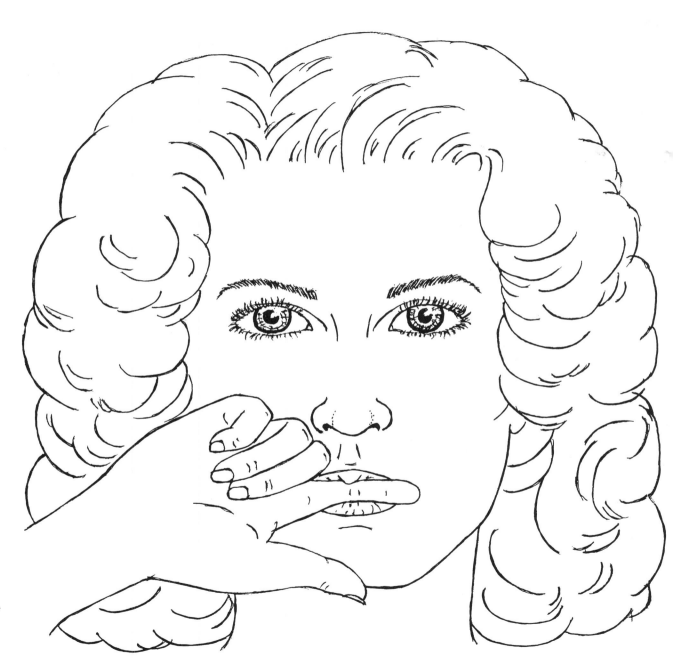

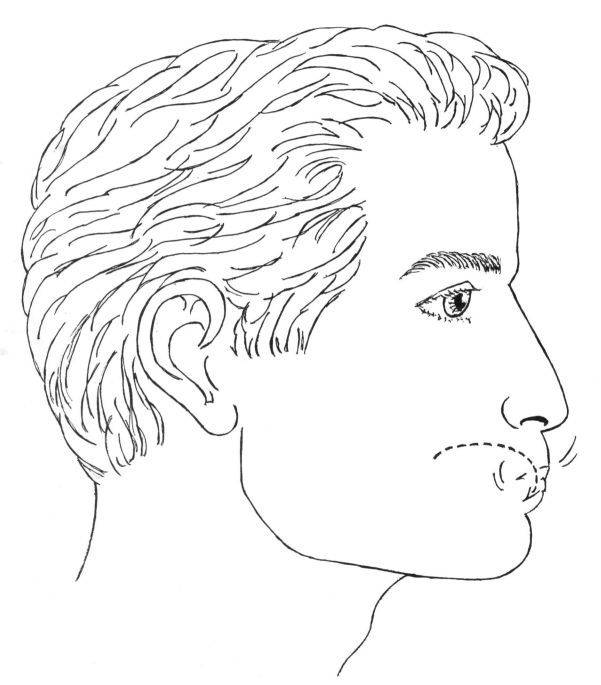

Exercise Three

1. Position the tongue so it points down and its tip is in front of your lower teeth.

2. Stiffen the tongue and keep your lips closed tight. Keep tongue stiffened and use it to resist the pressure of your lips.

3. Take a deep breath and tighten your closed lips against your tongue. Hold lips and tongue in resistance to a count of five and exhale.

Do exercise six times daily.

Exercise Four

1. Position the tongue so its tip is between your lips.

2. Press the upper lip downward against the tongue.

3. Stiffen the tongue so that it does not move when you press your upper lip down against it.

4. Hold tongue and lip in resistance to a count of three.

Do exercise six times daily.

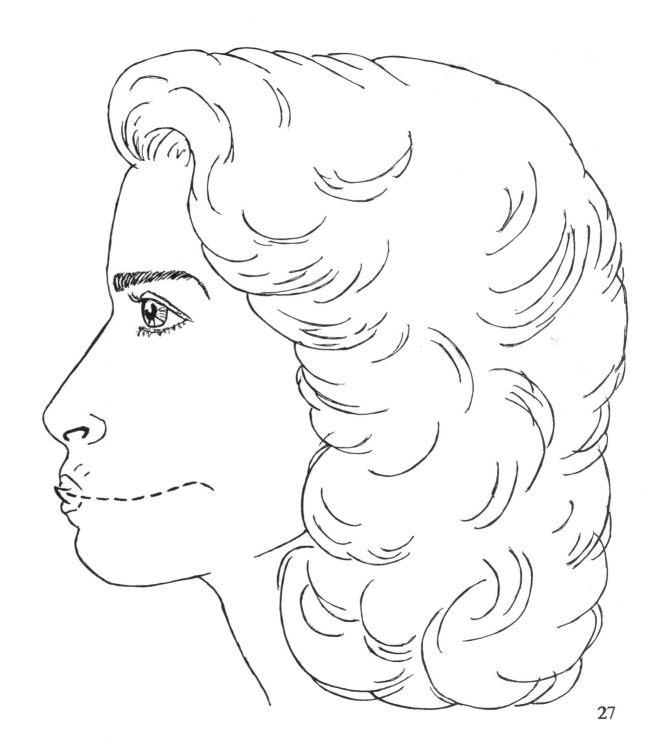

About Taking Deep Breaths

Breathing deeply insures that the muscles have an ample supply of oxygen in an exercise. However, if you experience dizziness, light headedness, or any other discomfort when you take the deep breaths called for, do regular breathing instead and take deep breaths only when your muscles need additional oxygen.

Exercises For
Women And Men Over 40

When we celebrate our 40th birthday, we enter a decade in which there is a tendency for looseness to develop in the skin of the face. This developing looseness calls for special preventive exercises for the lips and lower face.

The next three exercises were designed for you if you are over 40. They tighten the cheek, mouth, chin and jaw muscles.

The exercises involve placing the fingers inside the mouth and I don't recommend them for you if you are in your 30's and the skin of your lower face is still firm and tight. Although the risk of stretching the skin is very small, it is better that you practice skin safety and postpone doing the exercises until you have celebrated your 40th birthday.

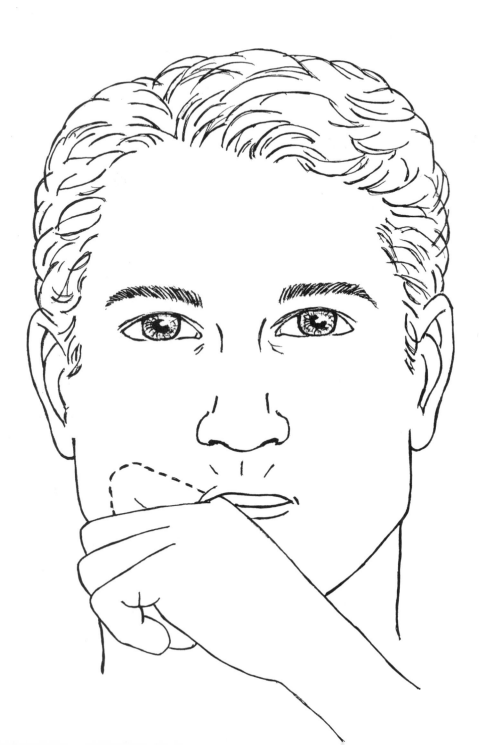

Over 40 Exercise One

For The Right Jaw Muscle

1. Position your left forefinger inside your mouth so the finger is under the right jaw muscle.

2. Take a deep breath and tighten the jaw muscle against the finger. Hold to a count of five and exhale.

For The Left Jaw Muscle

1. Position your right forefinger inside your mouth so the finger is under the left jaw muscle.

2. Take a deep breath and tighten the jaw muscle against the finger. Hold to a count of five and exhale.

Do exercise four times daily.

Over 40 Exercise Two

For The Right Cheek Muscles

1. Place your left forefinger inside your mouth so the first knuckle touches the cheek bone and is between your cheek muscles and right upper gums.

2. Take a deep breath and squeeze the cheek muscles tightly against the finger. Hold to a count of seven and exhale.

For The Left Cheek Muscles

1. Place your right forefinger inside your mouth so the first knuckle touches the cheek bone and is between your cheek muscles and left upper gums.

2. Take a deep breath and squeeze the cheek muscles tightly against the finger. Hold to a count of seven and exhale.

Do exercise six times daily.

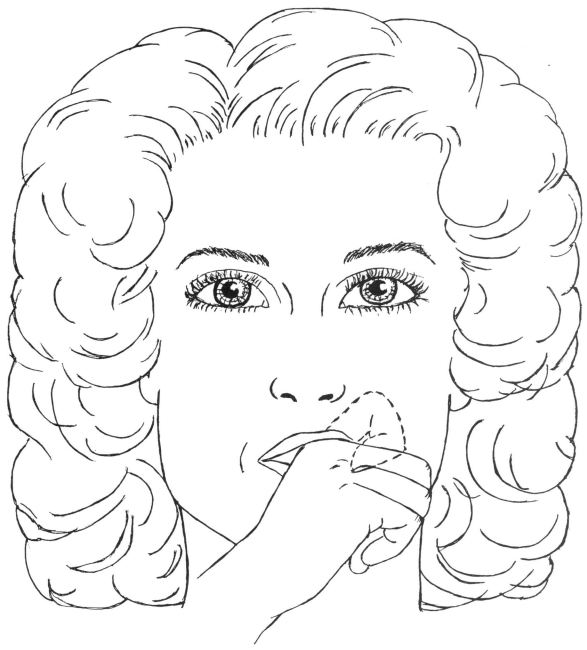

Over 40 Exercise Three

This exercise strengthens every muscle of the lower face. It contributes to fullness of the lips and it helps prevent hollows and sags in the contours of the lower face.

1. Position your two middle fingers between your lips so the fingers are directly under your nose and your finger tips are touching your teeth.

2. Extend your lips over your fingers as far as you can do so comfortably.

3. Inhale deeply and squeeze fingers tight with the mouth muscle. Squeeze hard and feel the mouth muscle tighten against the fingers.

4. Hold to a count of five as you exhale.

Do exercise twice in the morning, twice in the afternoon and three times in the evening.

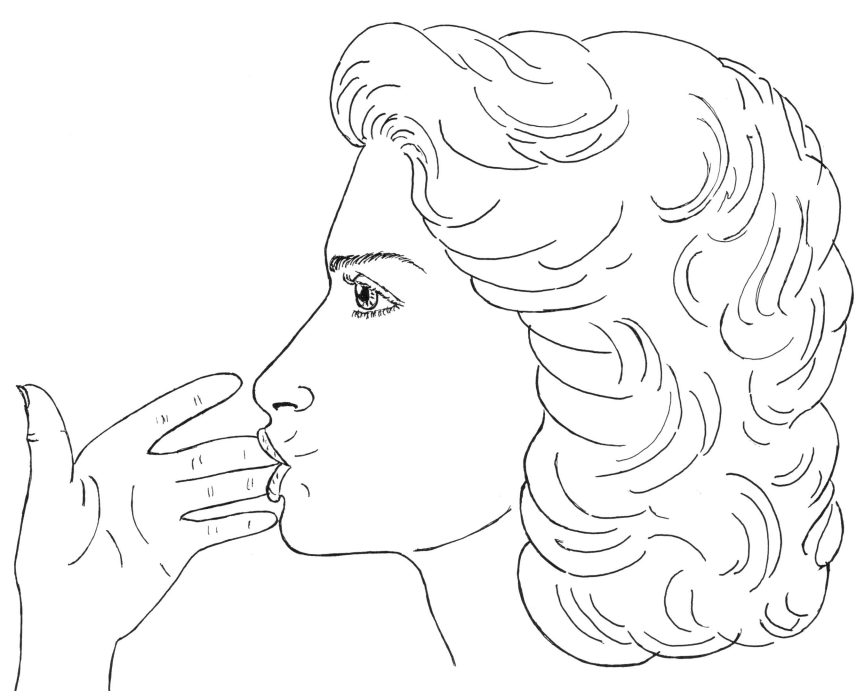

Designer Exercises For The Neck, Chin, Cheeks, Jaws, and Forehead.

The Swallow - An Exercise for the Neck

The Swallow tightens the muscles of the tongue and muscles of the inner neck.

One characteristic of premature aging is the bulge that develops in the front neck. This bulge forms when the tongue muscles get lazy and weak and allow the tongue to sink downward in the throat.

To see how this works, turn sideways in front of a mirror. With another mirror, look at your neck in profile and let your tongue relax and sink downward. Observe how the tongue's weight causes a bulge in the neck.

Now swallow and hold the tongue in the swallow position. This lifts the tongue high inside the mouth and presses it tightly against the top and back of the mouth.

The swallowing action tightens the muscles of the tongue and the muscles of the inner neck.

The Swallow significantly lessens the formation of a bulge in the neck.

Caution

The Swallow is an exercise that you can over-do. The goal of the Swallow is to retain or restore normal muscle strength but you don't want to over-tighten these muscles. Over-tightening will make it difficult for you to swallow food.

To guard against this, do the Swallow two times daily for one week and let seven days pass before you do the exercise again. In other words, do the Swallow daily every other week.

Important Safeguard

Monitor your ability to swallow food after you begin doing the Swallow. Be aware of each bite of food that goes down your throat.

If you find that you have any difficulty swallowing a bite of food, stop doing the Swallow for three weeks. When the tongue and inner neck muscles loosen and swallowing food is not interfered with by too-tight muscles, you can safely begin doing the exercise again.

The Swallow

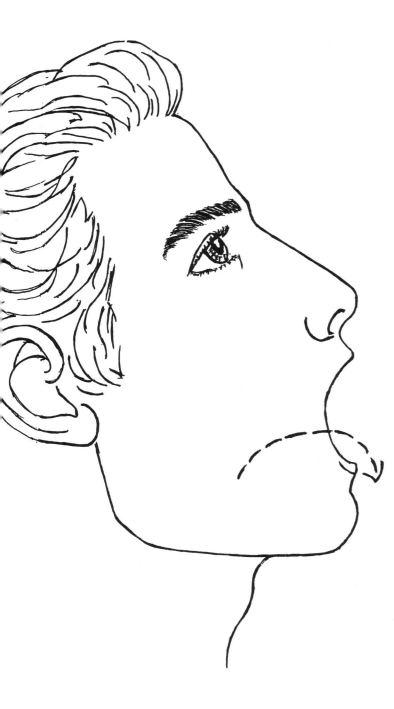

1. Tilt your head back and stick your tongue out and down over your chin.

2. Hold your tongue extended downward to a count of two.

3. Relax your tongue, tilt your head back and swallow.

4. Hold tongue in swallow position, pressed tight against the top and back of your mouth. Hold to a count of three.

Relax tongue and breathe deeply.

Do the swallow two times daily for one week. Then let seven days pass before you do the exercise again.

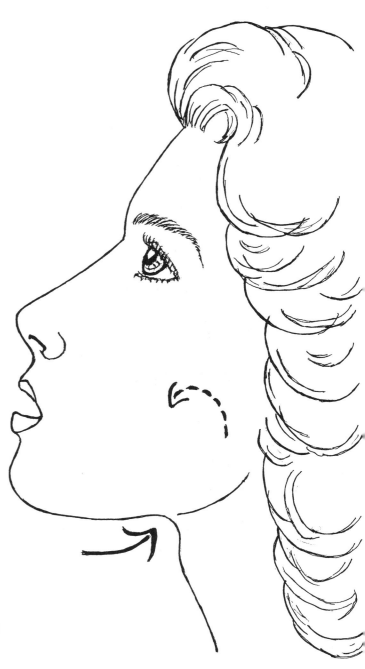

Exercise for the Outer Muscles of the Neck

1. Fill a 32 oz soft plastic bottle full of water.

2. Lie on the floor and balance the bottle on your forehead with your hands.

In the illustration the model is holding the bottle with one hand but it works better if you use both hands.

3. Hold the bottle in place with your hands and raise your head at least 1/4 inch off the floor.

4. Use your outer neck muscles to hold your head off the floor to a count of three.

Relax and Breathe deeply.

Do Exercise Five Times Daily.

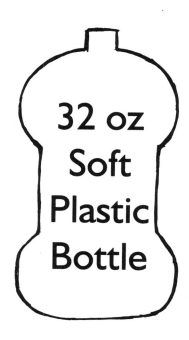

32 oz Soft Plastic Bottle

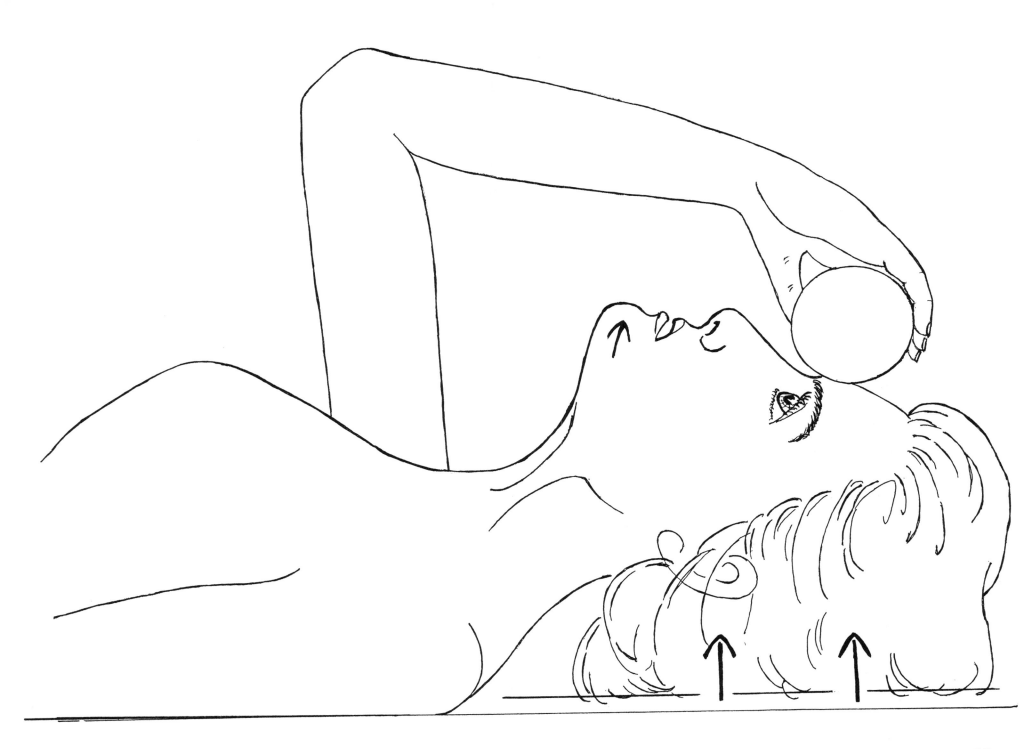

Exercises for the Muscles of the Eyes, Cheeks and Forehead.

In the next three exercises you will use the muscles to squeeze your eyelids together, to squeeze your eyebrows downward, and to squeeze your cheeks upward.

Normally these muscle actions would make lines and creases in the skin. This won't happen because the exercise is designed so your hands prevent most of the movement in the skin when the muscles contract.

The heels of your hands fit naturally into your eye sockets and when the heels and palms of the hands resist the muscle contractions, this forces the muscles to work harder.

When the muscles work harder, they grow stronger and increase in size. This increase in strength and size provides better support for the overlying skin.

Exercise One

1. Place your hands over your closed eyes so the heels of your hands rest gently against your eyelids.

2. Let the sides of your hands rest against the skin between your eyebrows. Let your little fingers rest against your center forehead.

3. Squeeze your eyelids together tightly as you take a deep breath.

Let your hands provide a gentle resistance that forces the muscles to work harder. Hold the muscles squeezed tightly to a count of five as you exhale.

Do Exercise Three Times Daily.

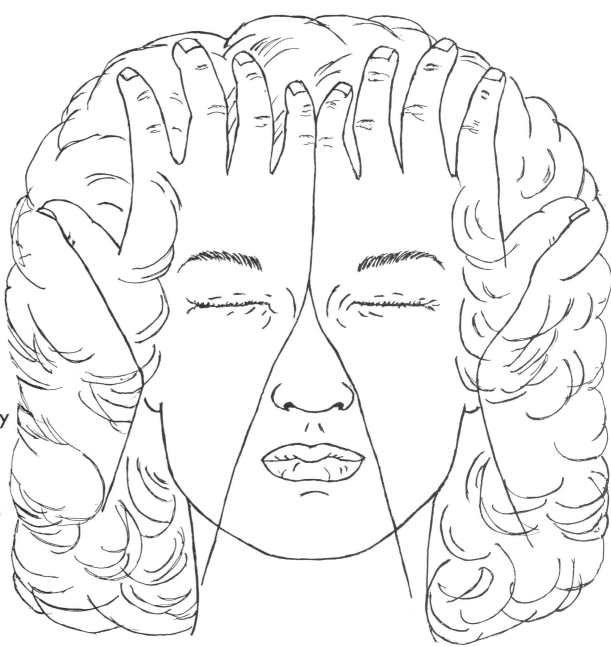

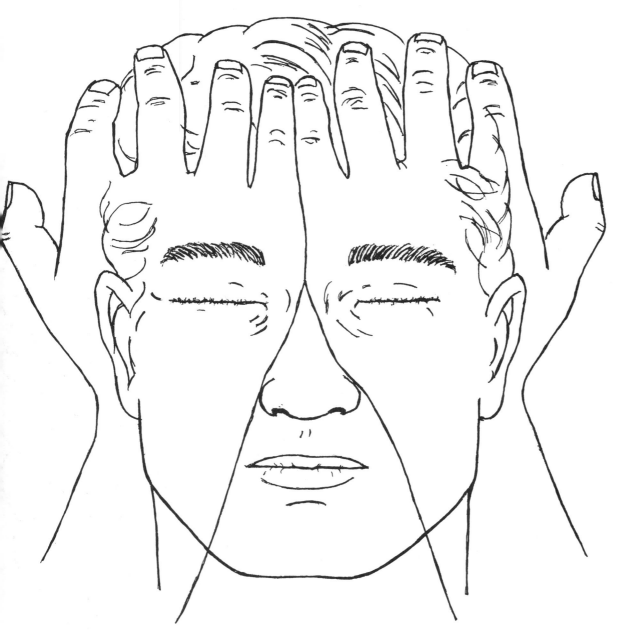

Exercise Two

1. Rest your hands gently against your closed eyes.

2. Let your hands rest firmly against the skin of your forehead.

3. Squeeze your eyebrows downward against the resistance of your hands as you take a deep breath.

Feel your hands provide resistance that makes the forehead muscle work harder.

Hold resistance to a count of five and relax.

Do Exercise Twice Daily.

Exercise Three

1. Rest your hands gently against your closed eyes.

2. Let the lower hands rest against your cheek bones.

3. Squeeze your cheeks upward against your hands.

Feel your hands provide a gentle resistance that makes the cheek muscles work harder.

Hold resistance to a count of five and relax.

Do Exercise from Two to Four Times Daily.

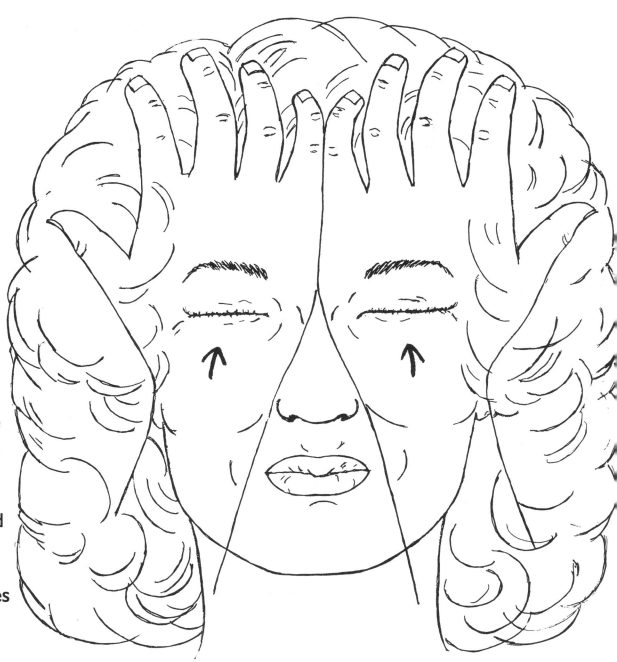

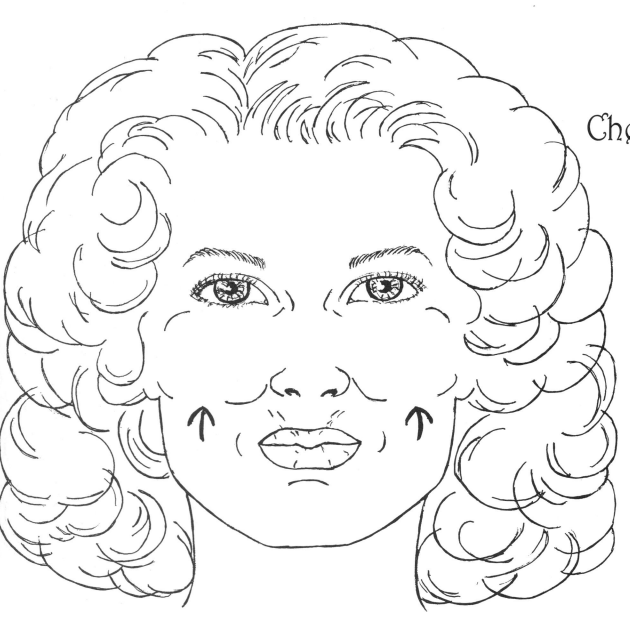

Cheek Muscle Tightener

1. Take a deep breath, close lips and tighten the corners of the lips against your teeth.

2. Focus the tension in the cheeks where the arrows point.

3. Widen the tension upward into the cheeks so you can feel the cheek muscles tighten against the cheek bones.

Hold the tension to a count of three and exhale.

Do Exercise Three Times Daily.

Jaw Muscle Tightener

1. Take a deep breath, close lips, and tighten the corners of the lips against your teeth.

2. Focus the tension in the jaw muscles where the arrows end and tighten your jaw muscles against your teeth.

Hold to a count of three and exhale.

Do Exercise Three Times Daily.

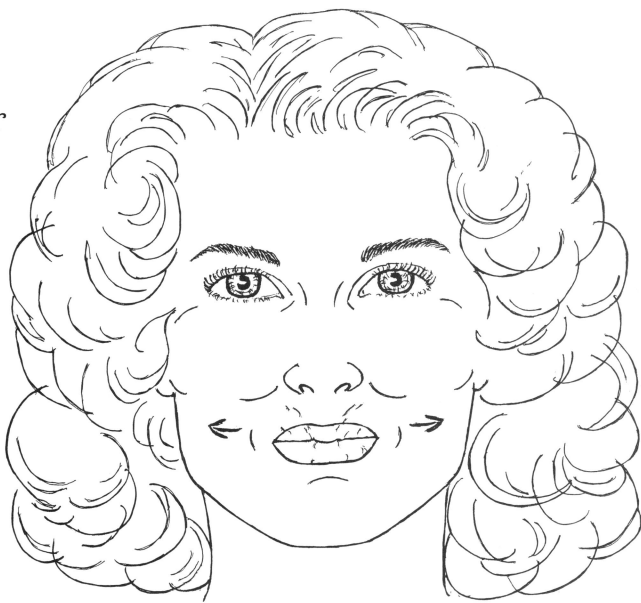

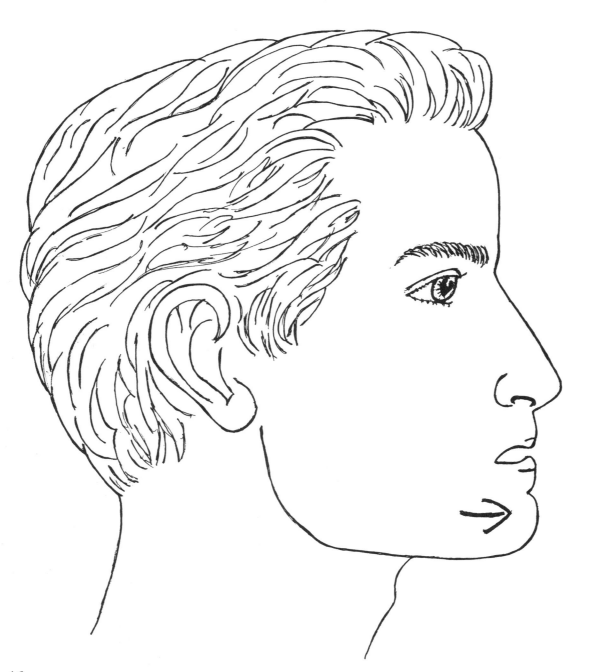

Chin Firming Exercises

Exercise One

1. Push your chin forward and tighten the chin muscles as you take a deep breath.

Lips can be closed or slightly parted.

2. Hold tightening of the muscles to a count of six.

Exhale and relax.

Do Exercise Three Times Daily.

Exercise Two

1. Tilt your head backward and push your chin forward. Tighten the chin muscles as you take a deep breath.

2. Hold the tightening of the muscles to a count of four.

Exhale and relax.

Do Exercise Three Times Daily.

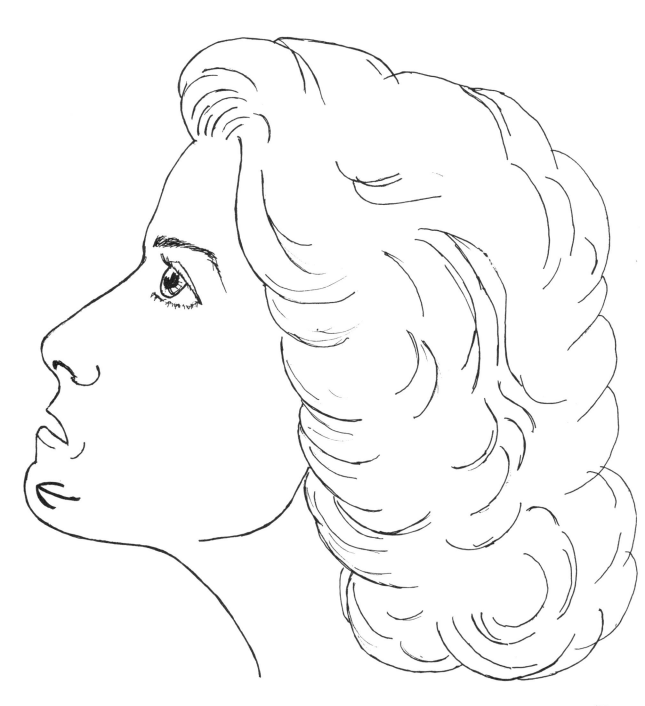

Skin Firming Exercises

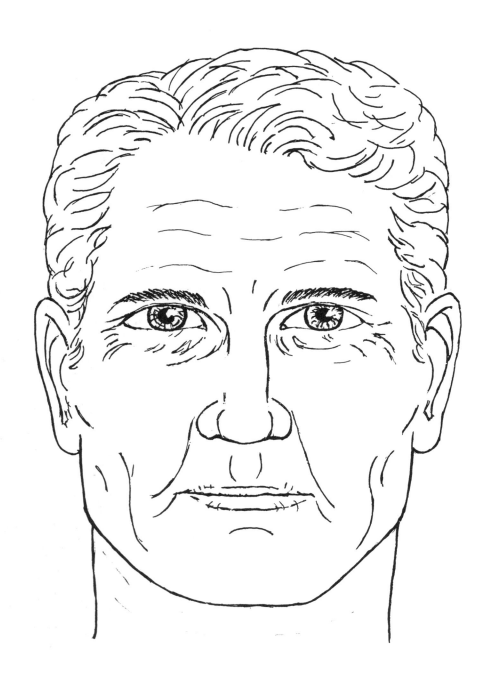

Skin Firming Exercises

Help Prevent the

Face-Fallen Look.

This look is a

Premature Aging

Phenomenon that

Diminishes the

Beauty of the Face.

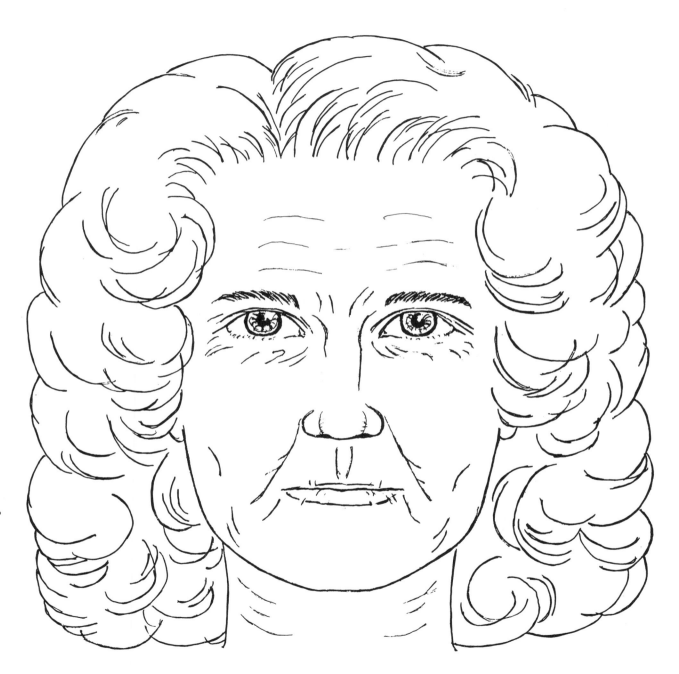

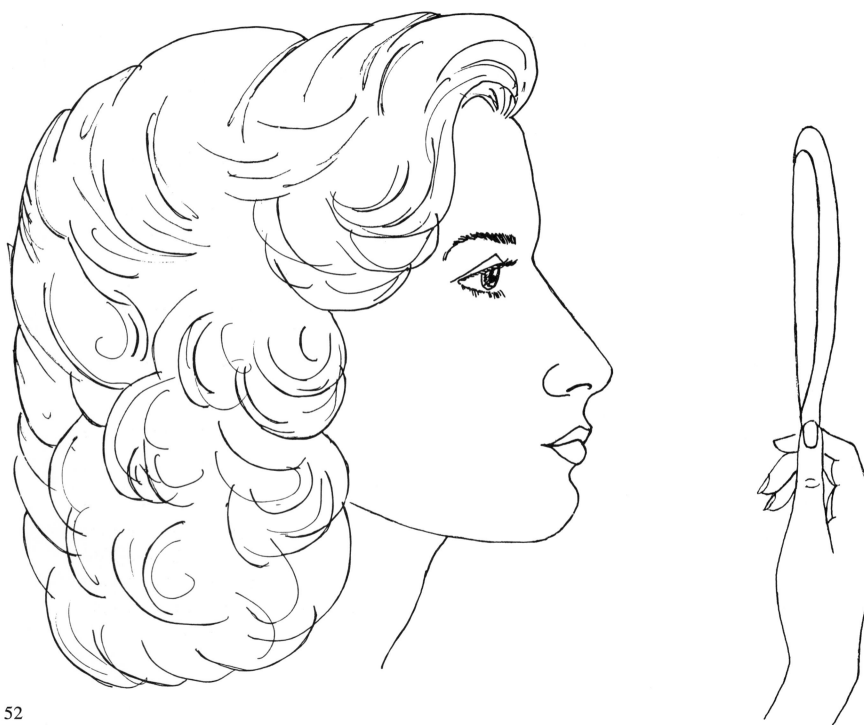

Skin-Firming Exercises and Biofeedback

After everybody's 30th birthday, the skin becomes less firm because it begins losing some of the support of facial muscles; the muscles are being weakened by the premature aging process. Skin-firming exercises strengthen and tighten these muscles.

Educating the muscles of the face to do these exercises involves the use of biofeedback, a pleasant procedure used to train muscles to contract in beneficial ways.

Biofeedback subjects are usually linked to instruments that give them feedback on the muscles they are training; these instruments sometimes provide feedback in the form of tones or lights.

When you use biofeedback, you won't need sophisticated instruments; your mirror will give you the feedback you need.

The following biofeedback methods are used to train the muscles of the face:

1. Visual feedback from a mirror that lets you see what your muscles are doing.

2. Concentration that focuses your attention on the muscles.

3. Strong Will that adds determination to your effort to train the muscles.

These biofeedback methods are a combination of methods used by two pioneering biofeedback experimenters, Dr. Neal Miller and Dr. J. M. Blair. Both used biofeedback to train their muscles to do something the muscles normally could not do.

Dr. J. M. Blair's Experiment

Dr. Blair did the first recorded biofeedback experiment and it involved the muscles of the face. In 1901 he invented a machine that produced visual feedback. His goal was to find out if people could use their will to learn to control muscles they normally could not control. He worked with ears because people don't usually have the ability to make their ears move.

Blair linked his subjects to the machine which recorded even very small ear movements. Dr. Blair and his subjects tensed the muscles around the mouth and in the forehead and watched the machine's feedback as they tried to create ear movements by using the will.

They were successful. They had combined visual feedback with their will to train the muscles to contract in a way that moved their ears one at a time.

Dr. Neal Miller's Experiment

Almost sixty years after Blair conducted his experiment, Dr. Neal Miller decided to do an ear-wiggling experiment of his own. He had the ability to use his muscles to make both his ears wiggle at the same time and he decided to use biofeedback to train the muscles to wiggle each ear independently of the other.

Miller used his bathroom mirror for feedback and watched his reflection closely as he tried to get his right ear to move without moving his left ear. He imagined the left side of his head being numb and cold and he imagined he had feelings only on the right side of his head. Nothing worked until he tried concentration. By combining concentration and visual feedback from his mirror, Miller gradually gained control over muscles that moved his ears and he trained them to move his ears one at a time.

Training the Muscles - A Task
That Requires Time and Patience

Psychologists Miller and Blair were successful because they spent time patiently trying to get their muscles to do something the muscles normally could not do.

That is what you will be doing when you train your facial muscles to do skin-firming contractions. You will be educating your muscles to tighten in a way they normally cannot do.

Trying Is Training

In each training exercise you will be trying hard to get your face muscles to do skin-firming contractions and it is your trying effort that trains the muscles.

Time Required

If you do the training exercises for at least fifteen minutes every day, you will have your muscles trained to do skin-firming exercises in about three weeks.

However, you may find that your facial muscles require less than three weeks to be trained or you may find that they require a longer training period.

Devote whatever time you need to teach your muscles to do skin-firming exercises. Firming the skin is a valuable skin-care technique and worth the time you spend learning how to accomplish it.

Training Exercises

Information About the First
Two Training Exercises

Squint lines under the eyes are usually the first visible signs of premature aging. Because of this, the first two training exercises teach the eye muscles to do skin-firming contractions. A squint contraction pulls the under-eye skin inward toward the nose; the skin-firming contraction pulls the under-eye skin in the opposite direction, away from the nose and toward the ear. A description of squints and squint consequences follows on the next two pages.

Squint Contractions

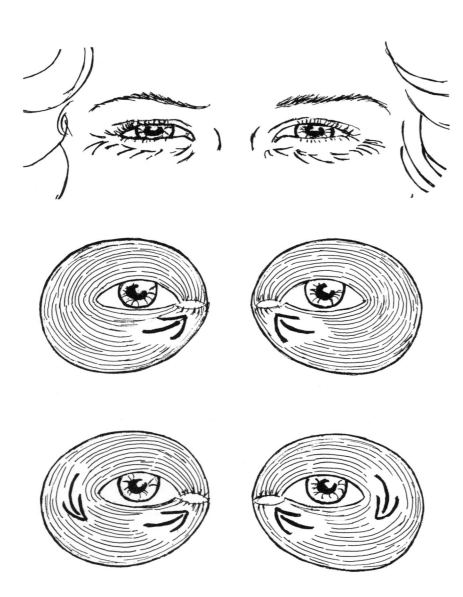

The under-eye skin is pulled into a squint thousands of times before the 31st birthday.

A squint contraction pulls the under-eye muscle toward the nose and the skin attached to the muscle is pulled along with it.

Since the eye muscle is circular, a squint exerts a downward pull on the muscle above the eye. This pull is slight but it has a loosening effect on the skin above the eye.

Squint Consequences

The thousands of pulls on the skin result in squint lines and hollows around the eyes. Eventually, bags under the eyes can form.

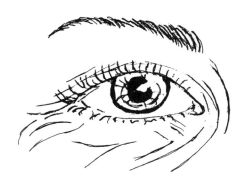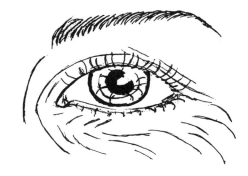

The first two exercises train the eye muscles to do a skin-firming exercise that counteracts the premature aging effects of squinting. The primary purpose of the exercises is to firm the under-eye skin, but they also have a firming effect on all the skin around the eyes.

Training the Eye Muscles to do Skin Firming Exercises

Training Exercise One - The Eyelid Lift

Your goal in this exercise is to train each eye muscle to do the Eyelid Lift, a muscle action that lifts the lower eyelid without squinting. Visual feedback from your mirror, Concentration, and Will are your training tools.

Remember, the Will is a conscious signal you send from your brain to a muscle when you want the muscle to do something for you.

Training the Right Eye Muscle

1. Visual Feedback from Mirror
Squint hard three times with both eye muscles and observe how the squints raise the lower eyelids.

Open your eyes as wide as you can and hold to a count of four. Do this three times.

Press your lips flat together and pull them inward with suction as you look closely in your mirror. Find a tiny spot of skin under your right eye in the same location as the circle in the illustration. Visualize the muscle fibers under the skin.

2. Concentration
With eyes opened wide, stare hard at the tiny spot of skin and concentrate on it intensely.

You do not have to limit your concentration to one spot of skin. You can choose other areas in the under-eye skin at which you can direct strong, intense concentration.

3. Will
Start to squint with the right eye muscle, but only start. When the muscle begins to pull the skin toward your nose, stare harder and harder at the skin and try to make the muscle lift the eyelid without squinting.

Use determined will and strong concentration constantly as you train the muscle.

Do this exercise five times daily.

— — — — — — — — —

Training the left eye muscle

Follow the instructions for training the right eye muscle and substitute LEFT for RIGHT in each step of the instructions.

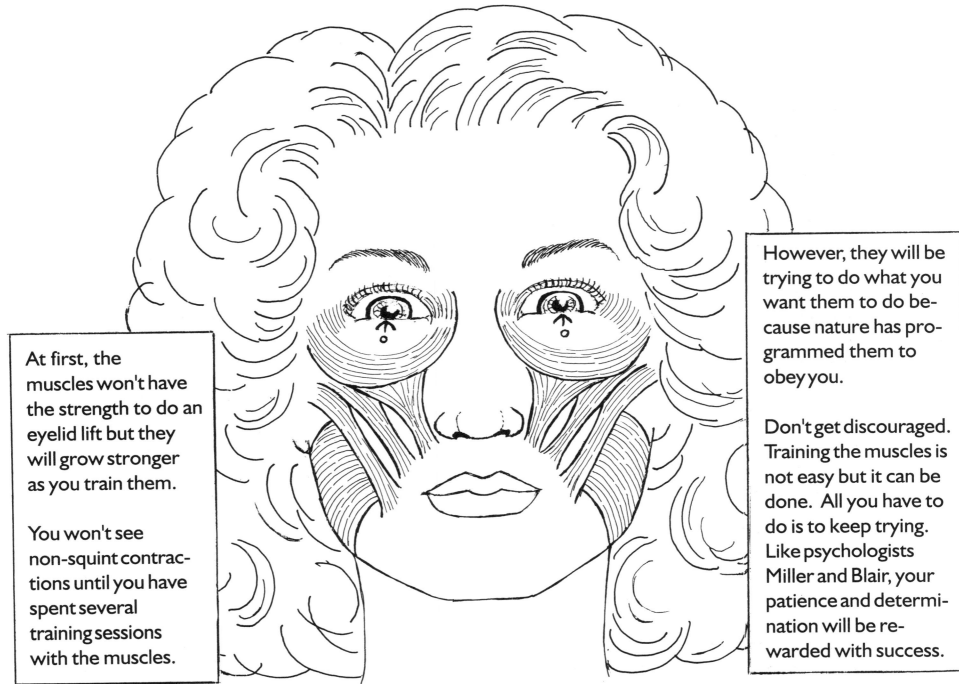

At first, the muscles won't have the strength to do an eyelid lift but they will grow stronger as you train them.

You won't see non-squint contractions until you have spent several training sessions with the muscles.

However, they will be trying to do what you want them to do because nature has programmed them to obey you.

Don't get discouraged. Training the muscles is not easy but it can be done. All you have to do is to keep trying. Like psychologists Miller and Blair, your patience and determination will be rewarded with success.

Training Exercise Two - The Reverse Squint

Your goal in this exercise is to train your eye muscles to do the Reverse Squint. In Reverse Squint action the eye muscles pull the under eye skin away from the nose and toward the side of the face. This reverse muscle action makes it difficult for squint lines to form and it minimizes squint lines that have already formed.

Training the Right Eye Muscle

Warm up the muscle by doing the Eyelid Lift.

During the exercise keep your eyebrows raised high, your eyes opened wide, and your lips pulled inward with suction.

1. Visual Feedback
Look in your mirror and focus on a tiny spot of skin under your right eye in the same location as the circle in the illustration.

Do the Eyelid Lift with the right eye muscle and hold in place as you continue.

Visualize the muscle pulling the spot of skin toward your right ear.

2. Concentration
Focus strong concentration on the spot of skin through a hard stare. The harder you stare, the stronger your concentration will be.

Try focusing your concentration on one or two different skin locations to see how they work for you.

3. Will
Combine determined will with strong concentration. Aim this powerful combination at the skin through a hard stare as you try to make the muscle do a Reverse Squint.

Do this exercise six times daily.

– – – – – – – – –

Training the left eye muscle

Follow the instructions for training the right eye muscle and substitute LEFT for RIGHT in each step of the instructions.

Although you won't see any reverse muscle movement at first, the muscle fibers are receiving your signals and they will be trying to follow your instructions.

The harder you try to do a Reverse Squint, the harder the muscles will try to do a Reverse Squint.

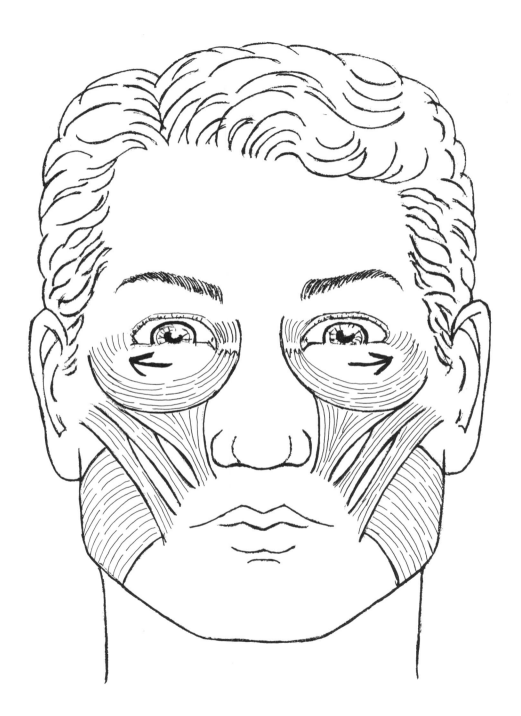

Pulling Your Lips Inward With Suction Gives The Eye Muscles Needed Resistance To Work Against.

Remember - Take deep breaths frequently to supply the muscles with oxygen. It works best if you take a deep breath at the beginning of each trying effort and exhale as you continue.

Cheek Muscle Training Exercises

Cheek Muscles and Skin-Firming Contractions

When Cheek Muscles one, two and three contract, they shorten upward toward the cheek bone. These contractions raise the upper lip using muscle fibers deep inside the cheeks; these fibers are too far from the skin's surface to have any beneficial effect on its appearance.

Skin-firming contractions are different. They are done with cheek muscle fibers near the surface of the skin. When these fibers contract, they don't raise the upper lip; they tighten the skin. Since the near-surface fibers of the cheek muscles are too close to the skin's surface to participate in the contractions that raise the upper lip, this leaves them with nothing much to do except get lazy and weak from lack of exercise.

Skin-firming exercises make these fibers grow stronger and increase in size. This helps prevent the flat look that can happen to the skin when it ages prematurely.

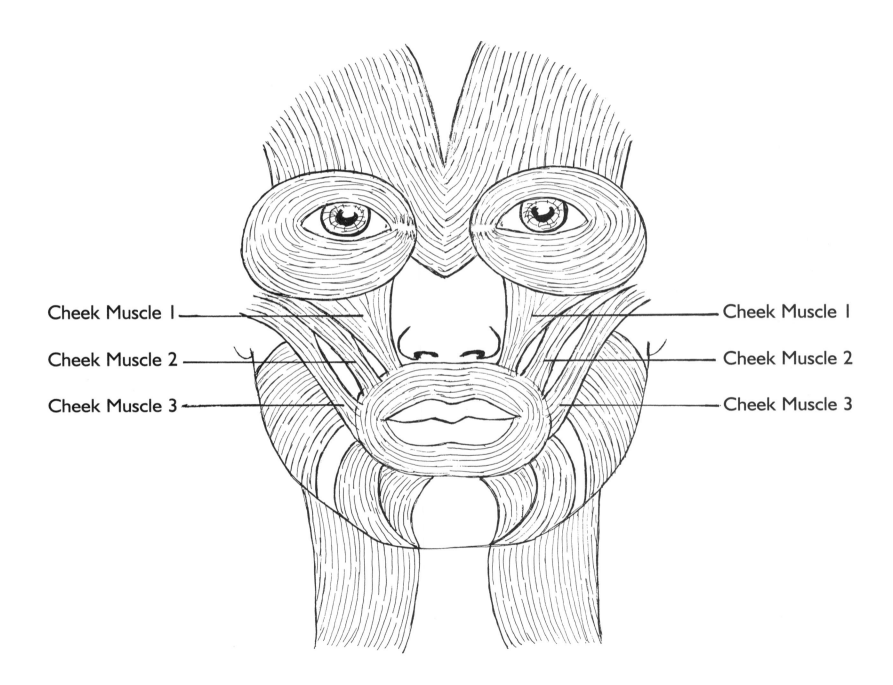

Cheek Muscle 1

Cheek Muscle 2

Cheek Muscle 3

Cheek Muscle 1

Cheek Muscle 2

Cheek Muscle 3

Training Exercise for Cheek Muscle One

Your goal is to train cheek muscle one to contract in a way that tightens itself and tightens the skin upward.

Training Right Cheek Muscle One

Throughout the exercise, keep your eyes opened wide, your eyebrows raised high, and your lips pulled inward with suction.

Do a Reverse Squint with the right eye muscle and hold it in place as you continue.

1. Visual Feedback
Look in your mirror and focus your attention on a small spot of skin in the same location as the circled spot in the illustration. It will be at the base of cheek muscle one, just above your smile line.

2. Concentration
Look in your mirror and stare hard at the spot of skin. Concentrate with intensity on the skin and visualize the muscle fibers shortening and pulling the skin upward.

- Keep lips pulled inward with suction.

3. Will
Combine strong, determined will with your concentration.

Stare harder and harder at the targeted skin and try to make the underlying muscle fibers contract upward.

Try for an upward movement in the skin for one full minute.

Do exercise five times daily.

— — — — — — — — — — — —

Training Left Cheek Muscle One

Repeat the training steps for the right cheek and substitute LEFT for RIGHT in each step.

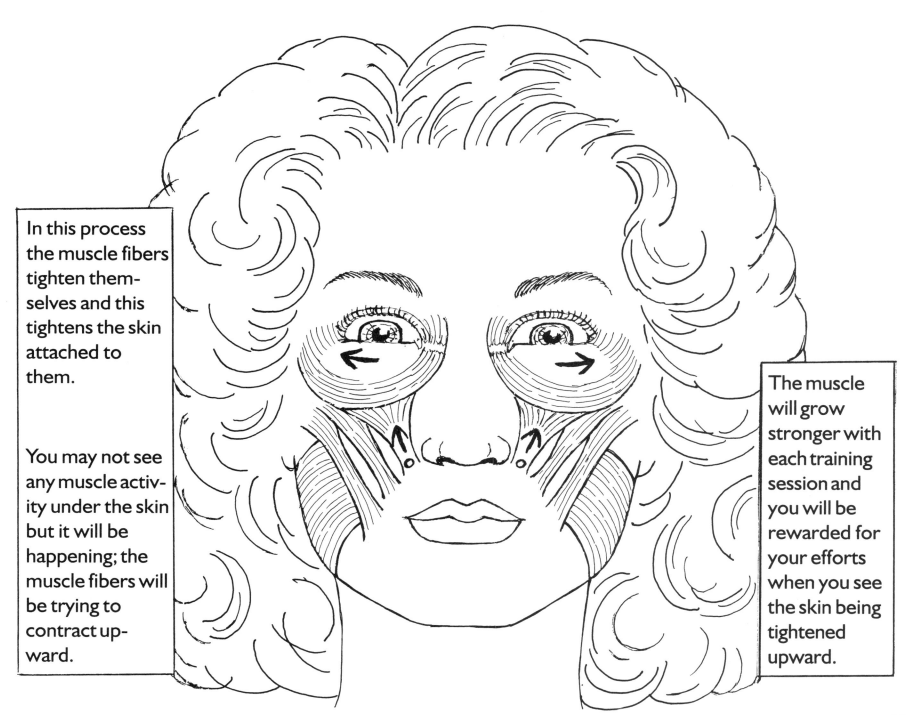

In this process the muscle fibers tighten themselves and this tightens the skin attached to them.

You may not see any muscle activity under the skin but it will be happening; the muscle fibers will be trying to contract upward.

The muscle will grow stronger with each training session and you will be rewarded for your efforts when you see the skin being tightened upward.

73

Training Exercise for Cheek Muscle Two

Your goal is to train cheek muscle two to contract in a way that tightens itself and tightens the skin.

Training Right Cheek Muscle Two

Throughout the exercise, keep your eyes opened wide, your eyebrows raised high, and your lips pulled inward with suction.

Do a Reverse Squint with the right eye muscle and hold it in place as you continue.

1. Visual Feedback
Look in your mirror and focus your attention on a small spot of skin in the same location as the circled spot in the illustration. It will be at the base of cheek muscle two, just above your smile line.

2. Concentration
Look in your mirror and stare hard at the spot of skin. Concentrate with intensity on the skin and visualize the muscle fibers shortening and pulling the skin upward.

3. Will
Combine strong, determined will with your concentration.

Stare harder and harder at the targeted skin and try to make the underlying muscle fibers contract upward.

Try for an upward movement in the skin for one full minute.

Do exercise five times daily.

— — — — — — — — —

Training Left Cheek Muscle Two

Repeat the training steps for the right cheek and substitute LEFT for RIGHT in each step.

Keep trying
until you see
a tiny upward
movement in
each circled
spot of skin.

A tiny upward
movement
means you have
succeeded.

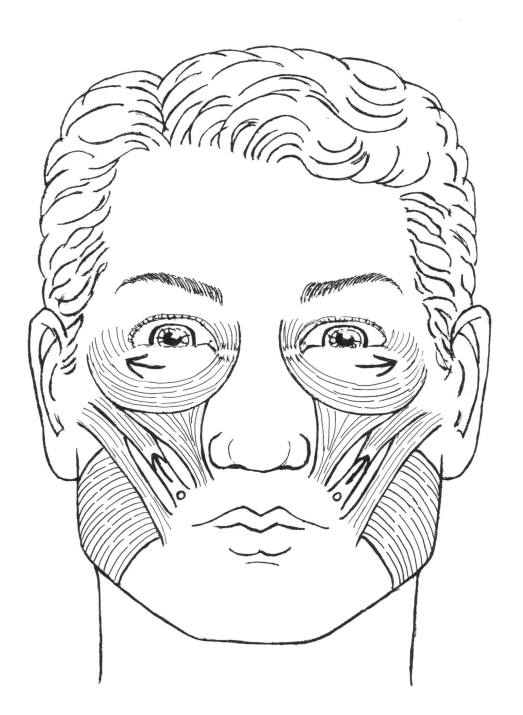

In this process
the muscle fibers
tighten them-
selves and this
tightens the skin
attached to
them.

As the muscle
grows stronger,
its fibers will
grow larger. This
increase in size
helps prevent
the formation of
hollows and lines
in the skin.

Training Exercise for Cheek Muscle Three

Remember, your goal is to train the cheek muscle to contract in a way that tightens itself.

Training Right Cheek Muscle Three

Throughout the exercise, keep your eyes opened wide, your eyebrows raised high, and your lips pulled inward with suction.

Do a Reverse Squint with the right eye muscle and hold it in place as you continue.

1. Visual Feedback
Look in your mirror and focus your attention on a small spot of skin in the same location as the circled spot in the illustration. It will be at the base of cheek muscle three, just above your smile line.

2. Concentration
Look in your mirror and stare hard at the spot of skin. Concentrate with intensity on the skin and visualize the muscle fibers shortening and pulling the skin upward.

3. Will
Combine strong, determined will with your concentration.

Stare harder and harder at the targeted skin and try to make the underlying muscle fibers contract upward.

Try for an upward movement in the skin for one full minute.

Do exercise five times daily.

_ _ _ _ _ _ _ _ _ _ _ _ _ _

Training Left Cheek Muscle Three

Repeat the training steps for the right cheek and substitute LEFT for RIGHT in each step.

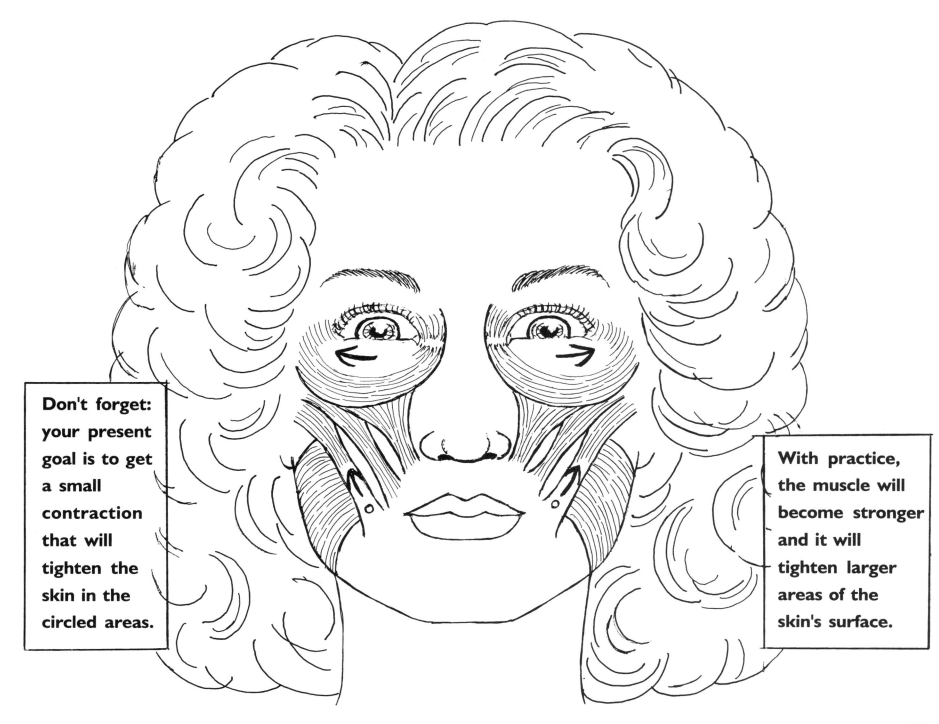

Don't forget: your present goal is to get a small contraction that will tighten the skin in the circled areas.

With practice, the muscle will become stronger and it will tighten larger areas of the skin's surface.

Advanced Training of the Cheek Muscles

Training the Right Cheek Muscles

1. Visual Feedback

Look in your mirror and focus your attention on three tiny spots of skin on your right cheek that are in the same location as the circles in the illustration.

These spots of skin will be just above your smile line.

2. Concentration

Do a Reverse Squint with the right eye muscle and hold it in place as you continue the exercise.

- Focus a strong stare at the three spots of skin.

- Take a deep breath and concentrate with increasing intensity on the skin.

- Strengthen your concentration by staring harder at the skin.

3. Will

Take a deep breath and combine will with concentration and

- Stare hard at the skin as you try to make the muscle fibers pull the skin upward.

- Use determination as you try for a small upward movement in the three spots of skin.

- Stare harder and harder as you try for one full minute.

Do exercise five times daily.

— — — — — — — — —

Training The Left Cheek Muscles

Repeat the training steps for the Right Cheek Muscles and substitute LEFT for RIGHT in each step.

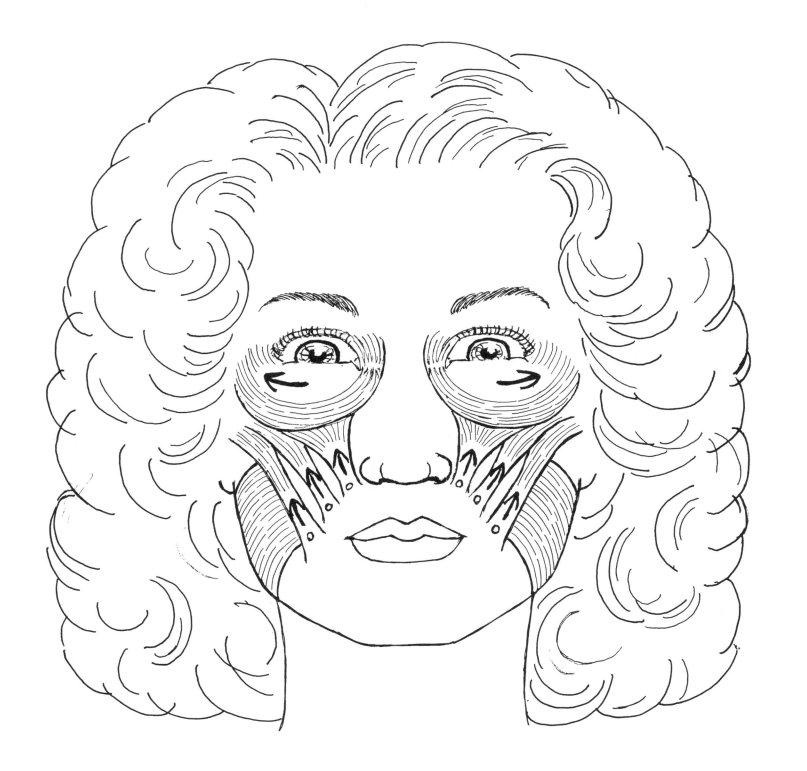

The training period for the eye and cheek muscles requires from one to three weeks of daily trying effort.

When your eye and cheek muscles have learned to do skin firming contractions, you are ready to go on to Skin-Firming Exercises.

Skin Firming Exercises I & II

Skin-Firming Exercise One

Right Cheek

Do a Reverse Squint with the right eye muscle. Hold the Reverse Squint in place as you continue the exercise.

1. Visual Feedback

Look in your mirror and focus your attention on three spots of skin on your right cheek that correspond to the three circles on the lower right cheek in the illustration.

2. Concentration

Focus an intense stare on the three spots of skin. Send your concentration through your stare to the skin and the underlying muscle fibers.

3. Will

Combine your will and concentration and visual feedback.

- **Use this powerful combination to make the muscle fibers tighten themselves and tighten the skin upward.**

Do exercise six times daily.

Left Cheek

Repeat the exercise steps for the Right Cheek and substitute LEFT for RIGHT in each step.

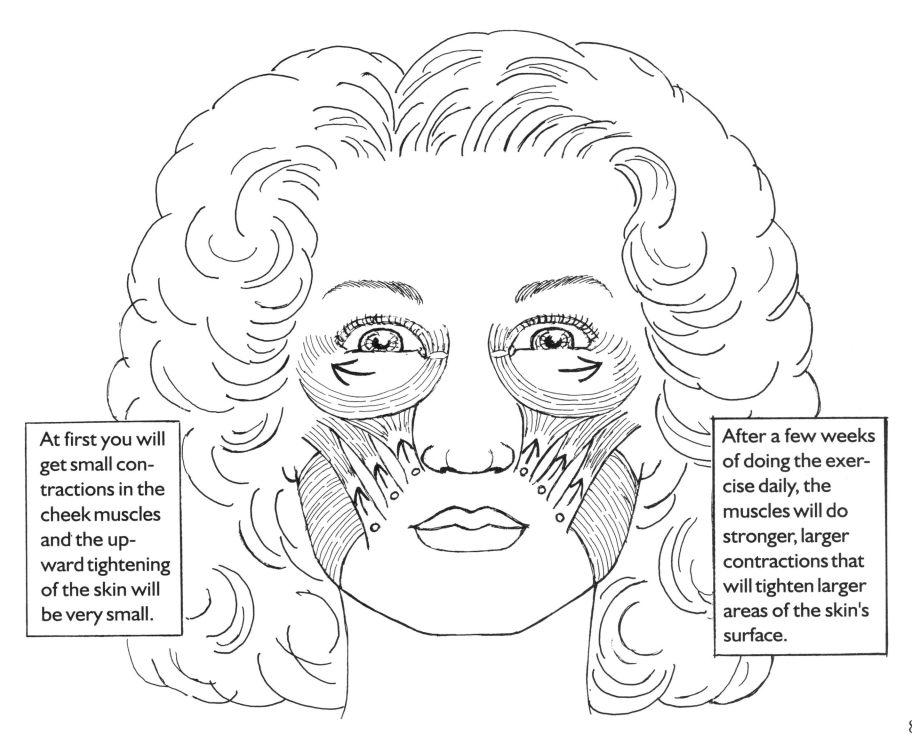

At first you will get small con-tractions in the cheek muscles and the up-ward tightening of the skin will be very small.

After a few weeks of doing the exer-cise daily, the muscles will do stronger, larger contractions that will tighten larger areas of the skin's surface.

Skin-Firming Exercise Two

Muscles are intelligent and they are great communicators. When one muscle learns how to do something, it communicates its knowledge to neighboring muscles. For example, while you were training your cheek muscles, their neighbors, the jaw muscles, were receiving much of this training. In this exercise you will persuade your jaw muscles to join the eye and cheek muscles in skin-firming contractions.

Right Jaw

Do a Reverse Squint with the right eye muscle. Hold in place as you continue the exercise.

1. Visual Feedback

Look in your mirror and find a spot of skin on your right jaw that corresponds to the circled spot on the right jaw in the illustration.

2. Concentration and Will

Combine concentration and will and use them to make the right cheek muscles pull the cheek skin upward.

Hold cheek muscles in upward contraction as you look in your mirror and focus your attention on the targeted spot of skin on your right jaw.

Visualize the muscle fibers under the spot of skin shortening, then tightening the skin upward.

Look in your mirror and direct a hard, powerful stare at the spot of skin on the right jaw.

Direct strong concentration and determined will to the muscle fibers through your stare.

Make the jaw muscle fibers contract so there is an upward pull on the targeted spot of skin.

Do this exercise six times daily.

– – – – – – – – – –

Left Jaw

Repeat the steps for the right jaw and substitute LEFT for RIGHT in each step.

Your primary goal is to tighten the surface of your skin; skin firming exercises will do that for you. In addition, these exercises will do much more for your face.

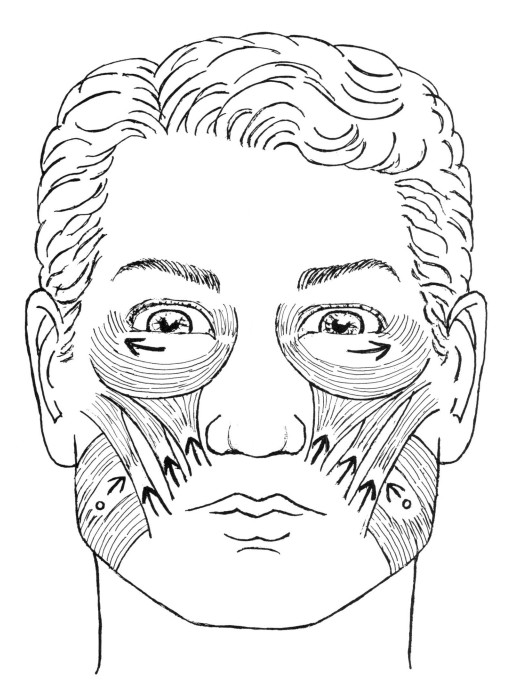

After you have been doing the exercises for about six months, fibers deep inside the cheeks and jaws will respond to your signals; they will tighten themselves and the tissues around them. This does much to firm the cheeks and jaws.

A Position That Gives You Gravity's Help

If you want gravity's help when you do Skin-Firming Exercises, lie on a flat surface with a pillow under your shoulders and neck.

Your cheek and jaw muscles will be able to do Skin-Firming contractions with less effort when you are in this position.

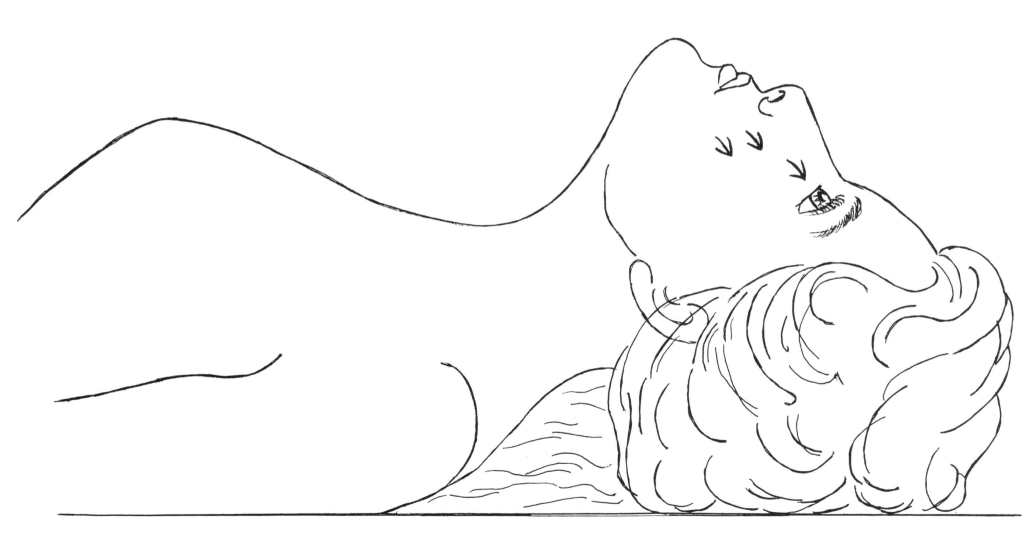

Bonus Section

Skin Smoothing Tape Masque for the Face and Hands

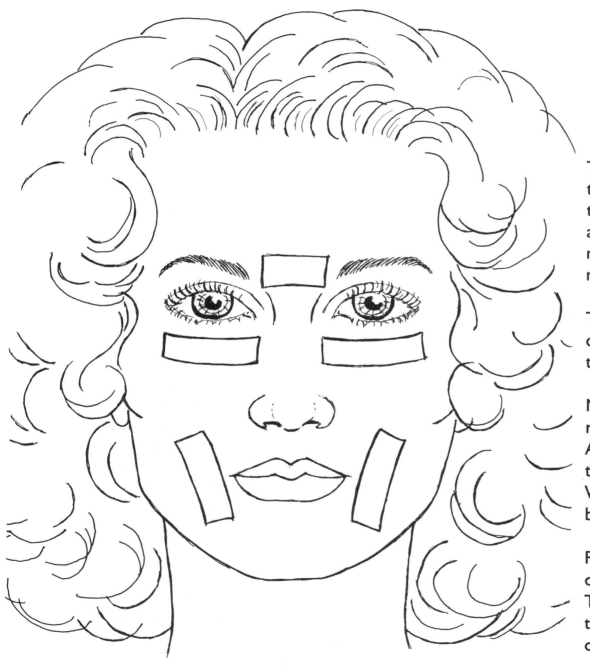

Introduction to the Tape Masque

The tape masque is composed of tape sections that cover skin areas most vulnerable to premature aging. The gentle pressure of the tape has a smoothing effect on the skin. It flattens puffiness, wrinkles, and lines and makes them less noticeable.

The masque is made of tape meant to be used on the skin. Surgical cloth tape, hypo-allergenic tape, adhesive tape or other tapes can be used.

Most of the tapes need some of their adhesive removed before they are placed on the skin. Adhesive removal is done by pressing tape to the forearm or to fabric one or more times. With some of its stickiness gone, tape can easily be removed from the skin.

Removal of the masque is done with a cosmetic cotton ball moistened with rubbing alcohol. The cotton is pushed under the edge of each tape; the moisture loosens the tape and it comes off the skin without causing discomfort.

The Tape Masque and Skin Safety

There are two things you need to do before using the Tape Masque.

1. Test Taping

Test taping enables your skin to adjust to wearing tape overnight. It is a total of twelve overnight wearings of selected tape sections. Instructions for test taping are on pages 92 and 93.

2. See your Doctor

Leading manufacturers of tape conduct skin safety tests in an effort to make sure their tape can be used on the skin with no harmful results. Nevertheless, it is important that you ask your doctor if you will experience any skin problems as a result of using the Tape Masque.

When you first begin wearing the masque, your skin may be pink and slightly chafed when you remove the tape sections or you may have a clogged pore in the skin. If either of these problems happen, postpone wearing the tape masque until the skin is clear.

Regular use of the masque causes the hair on the skin to break off and it slows hair growth to the extent that the skin has little hair on it after the masque has been used for a few weeks. You may be concerned about what will happen if you stop wearing the masque and the hair on the skin returns.

My own experience indicates there is no cause for concern. In the 15 years that I have used the tape masque, there have been times when I did not wear it for two or three months. The hair that grew back on my face and hands was the same in every way as the hair on my skin before I began using the masque. I have consulted with physicians about the possibility of unattractive hair regrowth after use of the tape masque and they tell me hair will grow back normally on a person's face after tape has been worn on the skin overnight.

However, your skin may be the rare exception and it is important that you ask your doctor if you will experience any adverse reactions from wearing the Tape Masque.

Test Taping

Use a moisturizer on the skin after removing the tape sections.

Rubbing alcohol is flammable. Do not use near open flame or electric heater.

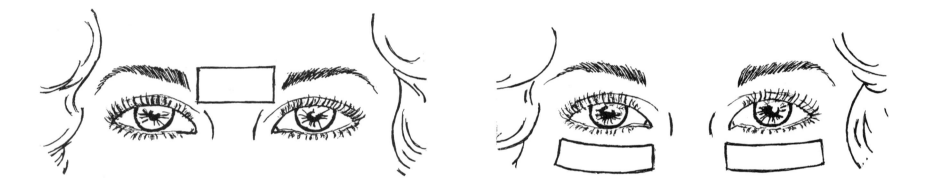

Step 1. Wear an adhesive-reduced tape between your eyebrows for one night. Remove tape with cotton ball moistened with rubbing alcohol.

Step 2. Wear an adhesive-reduced tape under each eye for one night. Remove tapes carefully with cotton ball moistened with rubbing alcohol.

Important!

Do the four test-taping steps at least three times before you go on to Tape Masque One.

This is a total of twelve overnight wearings.

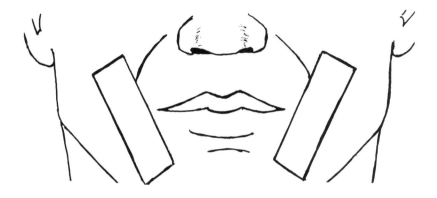

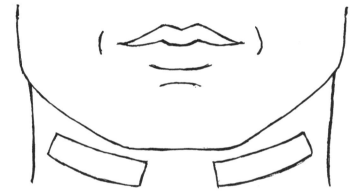

Step 3. **Wear an adhesive-reduced tape over each smile line for one night. Remove tapes with cotton ball moistened with rubbing alcohol.**

Step 4. **Wear an adhesive-reduced tape on each side of your neck for one night. Remove tapes carefully with cotton ball moistened with rubbing alcohol.**

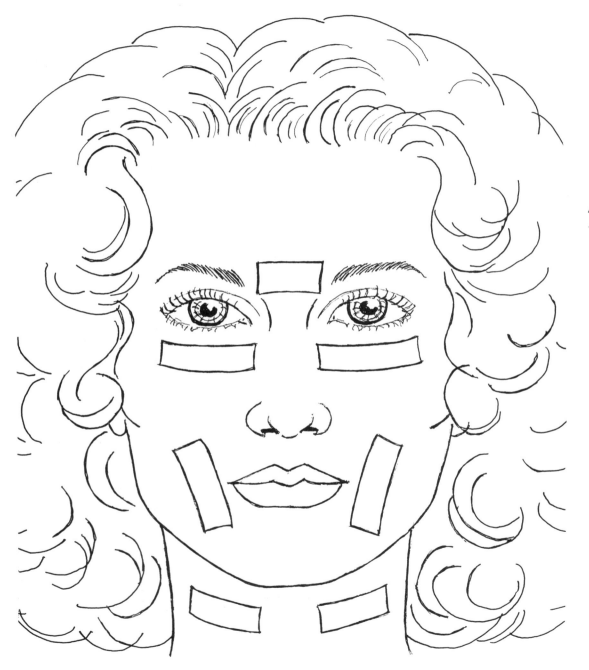

Tape Masque 1

Apply adhesive-reduced tape sections to your face and neck in the following manner:

1. Place a tape between your eyebrows.

2. Place a tape under each eye. Remove almost all the adhesive from these tapes before placing them. The under-eye skin is delicate and needs careful treatment.

3. Place a tape on each side of your lips and place a tape on each side of your neck.

4. Wear the tapes overnight and remove them with a cotton ball moistened with rubbing alcohol.

Wear this Masque twice a week for three weeks. If no skin problems develop, continue wearing the Masque until you want to cover more skin area with Tape Masque 2.

> Place tape sections on the skin with no pulling or stretching of the skin. The pressure of the tape does all the work for you.

Tape Masque 2

Tape Masque 2 is the same as Tape Masque 1 with the following changes:

1. Place two crossed tapes between your eyebrows.

2. Place an additional tape over each tape beside your lips.

Wear Tape Masque 2 twice a week for three weeks. If no skin problems occur, continue wearing this Masque until you want to cover more skin area with Tape Masque 3.

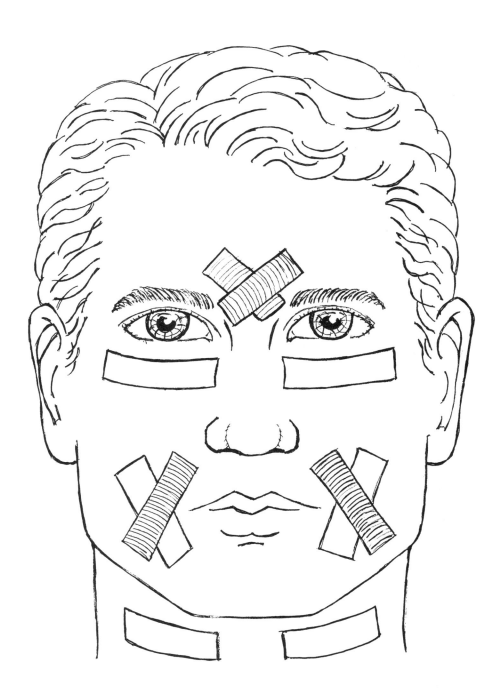

95

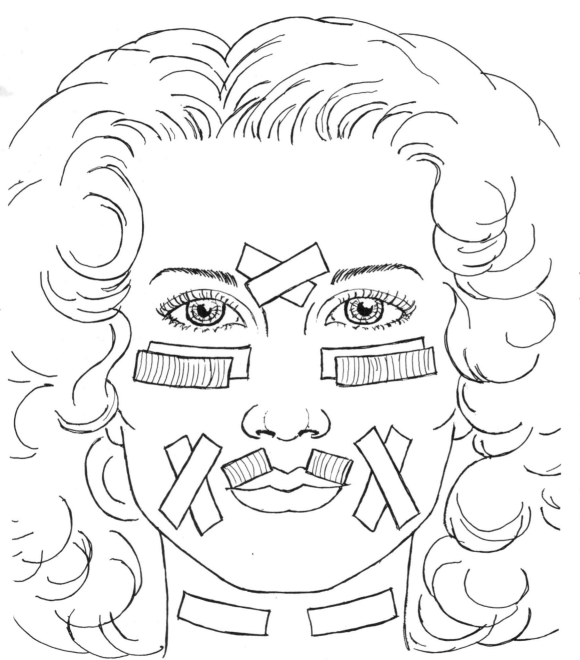

Tape Masque 3

Tape Masque 3 is the same as Tape Masque 2 with the following changes:

1. Place an additional tape over each tape under your eyes.

2. Place two tapes above the lips so they cover part of the upper lip line.

Wear Tape Masque 3 twice a week for three weeks. If no skin problems happen, continue wearing this Masque until you want to cover more skin area with Tape Masque 4.

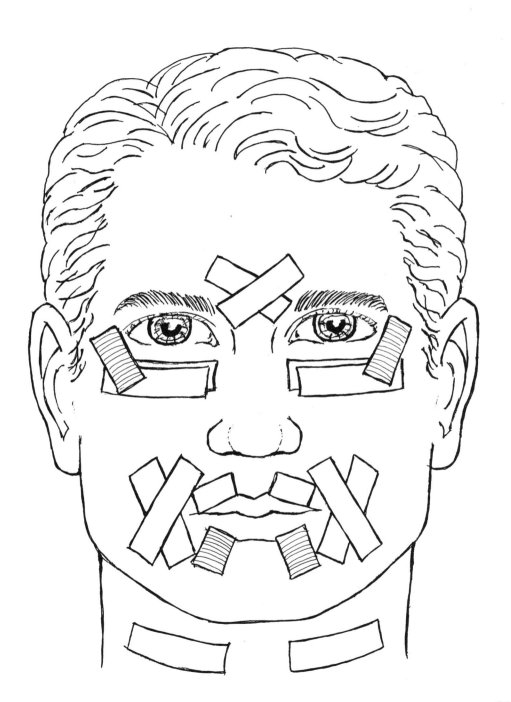

> If you have oily skin you will need to remove less adhesive from the tape.

Tape Masque 4

Tape Masque 4 is the same as Tape Masque 3 with the following additional changes:

1. Place a small tape beside each eye so that it extends over part of the under-eye tapes.

2. Place two tapes under the lips so they cover part of the lower lip line.

Wear Tape Masque 4 twice a week for three weeks. If no skin problems happen, continue wearing the Masque twice a week.

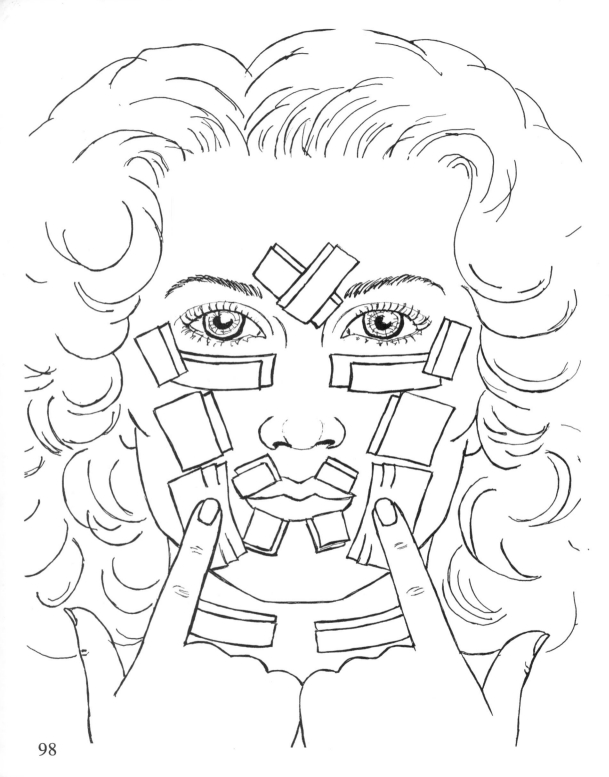

Tape Masque 5

Tape Masque 5 is designed to be worn after you have worn the first four masques for at least six months. This will give your skin time to adjust to overnight tape wearing.

This masque covers additional problem areas and each section has more than one layer of tape.

You can use extra tape layers in any area that needs additional pressure to keep the skin smooth.

Notice the three layers of tape beside the lips. Additional layers make the tape section stiff enough to hold an indention. If you use two or three tapes in this problem area, make an indention by pressing your finger to each tape when you apply it.

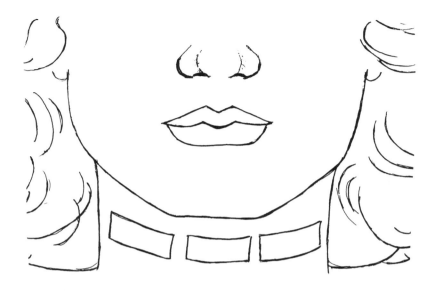

The neck area is delicate and sensitive to tape coverage. Go slowly if you want to cover more of the skin. Place tapes so there are areas of skin between the tapes; this allows the skin to breathe.

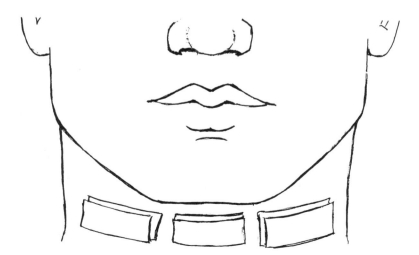

The five illustrated masques are meant to be tape arrangement guides. After your skin has adjusted to overnight tape wearing, you can use any tape arrangement that is right for you.

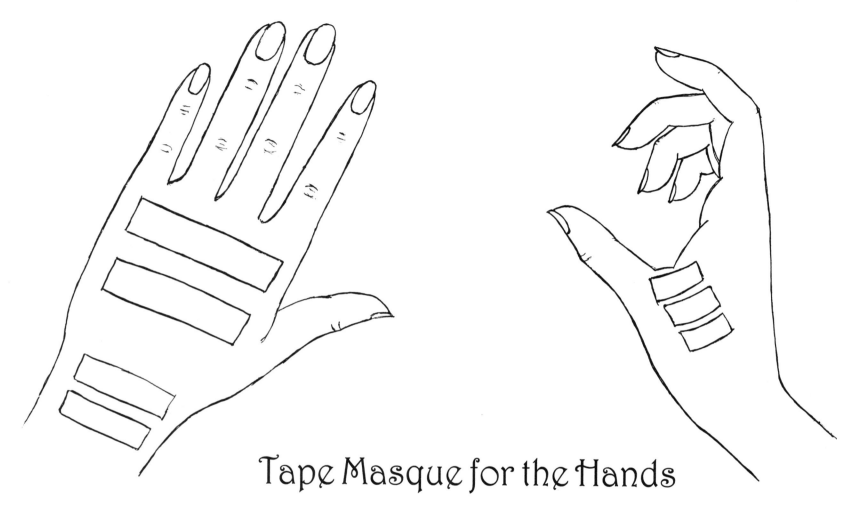

Tape Masque for the Hands

Test Taping

The skin of the hands is less sensitive to tape-wearing than facial skin but test taping is still needed.

To accomplish test taping, wear single layers of tape on the hands twice a week. Continue for three weeks.

Do some adhesive reduction before wearing the tapes.

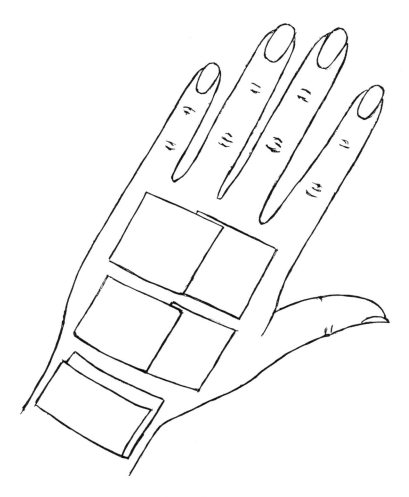
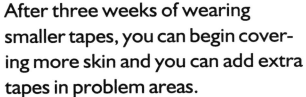
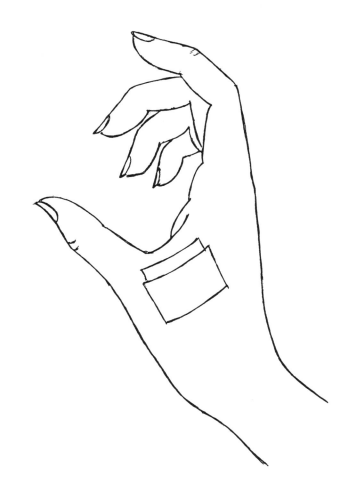

After three weeks of wearing smaller tapes, you can begin covering more skin and you can add extra tapes in problem areas.

The Tape Masque is designed to cover the skin where lines and wrinkles form. These areas include the wrists, back of the hands, and the skin at the base of the thumb and forefinger.

Wear the Tape Masque on your hands twice a week.

Bibliography

Edward VII and Queen Alexandra, A Biography In Word and Picture, Helmut and Alison Gernsheim, 1962, Published in Great Britain by Frederick Muller Limited.

The Prince & The Lily, James Brough, 1975, Coward, McCann & Geoghegan, Inc. New York.

Edward the Rake, John Pearson, 1975, Harcourt Brace Jovanovich, New York and London.

Edward VII, Prince and King, Giles St. Aubyn, 1979, Atheneum, New York.

Because I Loved Him, The Life and Loves of Lillie Langtry, Noel B. Gerson, 1971, William Morrow & Company, Inc., New York.

Edward & Alexandra, Their Private and Public Lives, Richard Hough, 1992, St. Martin's Press, New York.

The Jersey Lily, The Story of the Fabulous Mrs. Langtry, Pierre Sichel, 1958, Prentice-Hall, Inc., Englewood Cliffs, N. J.

Biofeedback and the Modification of Behavior, Aubrey J. Yates, copyright 1980, Plenum Press, New York.

Beyond Biofeedback, Elmer and Alyce Green, 1977, Delacorte Press/Seymour Lawrence.

Your Body and How it Works, Ovid K. Wong, Illustrations by Lindaane Donohoe, anatomical photographs by Lester V. Bergman & Associates, Inc., Childrens Press, Chicago, copyright 1986 by Regenstiener Publishing.

Man and His Body, The story of Physiology, Gordon McCulloch, 1967, Nature and Science Library, The Natural History Press, Garden City, New York.

A Biofeedback Primer, Edward B. Blanchard and Leonard H. Epstein, 1978, Addison-Wesley Publishing Company, Inc.

Biofeedback, Fact or Fad? Ann E. Weiss, 1987, Franklin Watts, New York/London/Toronto/Syndey.

New Mind, New Body, Barbara B. Brown, PH.D, 1974, Harper & Row, New York, Evanston, San Francisco, London.

Face Lifting Exercises, Molly Whisman, 1972.

Drawing the Human Head, Burne Hogarth, Watson-Guptill Publications, New York.

Principles of Anatomy and Physiology, Gerard J. Tortora and Sandra Reynolds Grabowski, 1993, HarperCollins College Publishers, New York.

Basic Physiology, Fred E. D'Amour. 1961. The University of Chicago Press.

Essentials of Human Anatomy, Russell T. Woodburne, 1978. Oxford University Press, New York, London, Toronto.

Athletic Training and Physical Fitness, Jack H. Wilmore, 1977, Allyn and Bacon, Inc., Boston-London-Syndney.

Shaping Up, George Mazzei, 1981, Ballantine Books, New York.